CONFESSIONS OF AN UNDERCOVER COP

Ash Cameron is a retired police officer, who worked in the undercover team in London. And that is all we can tell you.

ASH CAMERON

Confessions of an Undercover Cop

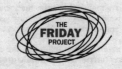

The Friday Project
An imprint of HarperCollins*Publishers*
77–85 Fulham Palace Road,
Hammersmith, London W6 8JB

www.harpercollins.co.uk

A Paperback Original 2013
1

Copyright © Ash Cameron 2013

Ash Cameron asserts the moral right to
be identified as the author of this work

A catalogue record for this book
is available from the British Library

ISBN 978-0-00-751508-0

Set in Minion by Palimpsest Book Production Limited,
Falkirk, Stirlingshire

Printed and bound in Great Britain by
Clays Ltd, St Ives plc

For Kenny.
And for our children.
See, we did have a life. Once.

The end

I was nineteen when I went to London to join the Metropolitan Police. I left the police force twenty years later, combining my leaving do with reaching forty.

They say life begins at forty. Mine didn't begin but it did change. I look back and wonder: that person, that police officer, was she me?

It's easy to see why cops feel battered when the people they deal with are often the bad people, the sick of mind people, and the victims and witnesses who are often distressed. And there are those who for whatever reason blame the police for everything.

Police officers can become embittered working in areas of high crime, populated by people with an abhorrent dislike of the law and those who try to enforce it. It's easy to understand the cynicism and jaded outlook when the days are filled with endless abuse and violence and grief. Even the officers working in the affluent suburbs and the beautiful countryside see people at their worst, all high drama and emotion, because in policing you are rarely involved with people at their best. After all, unless something's gone wrong, why would you need the police?

It's a strange phenomenon, and a bit perverse, when a good day at work can be a bad day, a sad day or a tragic day. Saving a life is one of those days.

There are also moments of fun and bizarre absurdity, slivers of sunshine, when you can laugh a real, gutsy belly laugh and know that today is one of the good days. They are golden.

I would have liked to reach the rank of inspector. Beyond that you become a manager, a pusher of pen and paper or mice and emails. Although the higher ranks are necessary, it's a totally different job. I finished my service as a detective sergeant and I was happy to settle for that, in the end.

Officers higher up the chain of command don't deal with the public. They deal with police officers and bureaucrats and forget what life is like policing the street. The real gutsy jobs are carried out by those who work hands-on with victims and suspects, getting down and dirty, and there are fewer hands-on officers nowadays, at a time when we need them more and more.

There are lots of opportunities in the police force. I wanted to experience as many as I could. I moved on, did different things, worked in diverse roles with different people in various departments. If I found myself grumbling too much, I knew it was time for change. I believe you make your own future and I've never sat around waiting for it to happen.

I've worked in the capital, in the East End, the West End, and north London. I've worked somewhere in the North too, in a constabulary. I've been a uniformed constable, an undercover cop, a detective and a sergeant. I've worked with the public in their many guises – victims, witnesses, prostitutes, rent boys, criminals, suspects, and many professionals in multi-agencies. I worked in London at the height of the IRA bombings and dealt with a few too. It's scary going to work knowing that you might be bombed at any time. As emergency workers, we'd run towards the explosion whilst urging everyone else to run away, and hoping there wasn't a secondary device primed to go off on our arrival. I've worked with the vulnerable, investigated racial incidents, homophobic attacks, elder abuse, missing people; I've worked in witness protection, on murder squads, in domestic violence and child protection. I've been a volunteer that took underprivileged kids on week-long camps. I've helped out in a women's refuge and come to the aid of Girl Guide and Brownie packs. I've saved lives and failed to save others. I've done some good things and I've also made mistakes, but I've always tried my best.

I had a fantastic time and have lots of marvellous memories. I miss the job incredibly, every single day. I loved it. All of it. Even when it was bad, it was good. It was part of me and it always meant more to me than perhaps it should have. It has taken a toll, like it does on every one of us who put everything we have into it. There are threats that still bounce around in my head from time to time, spat out by vile people who I helped to send to prison. I think they're probably out of jail now, and sometimes I feel them looking over my shoulder.

In the end, I had to make a choice. I could finish the last third of my career on completely restricted duties or take medical retirement due to a physical condition I was diagnosed with. It wasn't an easy decision and not the way I would have chosen to end my career, but I decided to leave with twenty years' service when there was a chance to start a different life while my children were young. I gave the job everything I had to give and I still believe the things I believed when I joined. I believe in justice, in right and wrong and, most of all, I still have that desire to help people.

It's a brave and frightening world out there, but leaving the police force was not the end of my life, even though at the time I wavered and thought it might be. I've had some wonderful, exciting and difficult times. When I left, many people asked what I was going to do. All I knew was I intended to take some time out, be a mum, keep my options open and see where life took me.

And I wanted to write, because ever since I could I have written stories and there are so many stories in my head.

These are my memories of all those things I've mentioned I did, and more. Not all of it is pleasant reading, but then not all of society is pleasant.

I wanted it all and I got a lot. These are my stories, told my way, with names changed to protect the guilty. And the innocent. A colleague might tell them differently.

In the beginning, there was light

All of the new recruits were sent to Hendon Police College. I was young, naive, and full of hope, anticipation and excitement, eager to complete the twenty-week residential course and get out onto the streets.

On the first day we had to swear our allegiance to the Queen. One hundred and sixty of us gathered together in the gym hall that I would come to hate during that twenty weeks.

A female chief inspector spoke, filling our heads with horror, some reality, a few romantic ideals, and a squiggle of 'What the hell have I done?'

'Some of you will stick the thirty years. The majority won't. You'll love it; you'll hate it. It won't always be pretty. I don't know anyone who hasn't been wounded on duty at least once, so be prepared. You might be injured and it could end your career. You might be shot. Stabbed. Killed. You will get hurt. Get used to it.'

She paused. 'Some of you won't make it through training school. Once on the streets you might decide you've had enough of being hated by the public, the press, the politicians and the prisoners, for you are nobody's friend. Remember that.'

My head spun. I looked at her. She was tough. I was soft. How would I cope with being hurt? Being hated? I only wanted people to think the best of me.

'But you may love it. It's the best job in the world when you save a life or stop a suicide. When you help people in the most difficult of circumstances. When you find a missing child and reunite him with a distraught family who feared the worst. But don't forget, you can be a hero one minute and then you're back out on the streets being pelted with flying bottles and vicious words.'

She looked around the room at the sea of fresh untainted faces in front of her.

'It's a good job if you can hack it. Not of all of you will. There are specialist departments to work in like mounted branch, dog section, CID, or undercover, so deep undercover that sometimes you forget who you are. You might decide to go for promotion. Or stay on the beat. Your whole time served might be in one police station, entrenched in a community. The rewards are there if you want them, but watch your back and those of your colleagues because they are the only allies you have.'

Among us were youngsters like me, not much in the way of life experience, starting out keen and vulnerable. There were others who'd decided they wanted a career change and policing had sounded like a good option, with a decent wage, job security and a pension. There were ex-service personnel who'd seen so much more already, and there were graduate entries straight from university.

We stood and listened and wondered why we thought we could do this job. The only dead body I'd seen was a boyfriend's grandmother in her coffin, but she had been over eighty and it didn't seem to count.

'You will come across things you don't like, things that turn your stomach, deal with offences you didn't know existed,' she continued. 'You will see things you know aren't right. You will have to decide what to do because when you're out there, you're on your own and only you can decide if you can live with the consequences. Only you are responsible for your actions.'

She was done. We filed out feeling like we'd been bollocked, looking anywhere but at each other lest we saw the fear.

In that moment I decided I could, I would do this job. If I survived training school . . .

Drunk and orderly

It's a well-known fact that policemen like to drink. It's one of those clichés found in crime novels and TV dramas. Like most clichés, it exists because there's a truth in there somewhere.

When I joined the Met, I didn't drink alcohol. I'd had the odd shandy, a couple of lager tops, a rare lager and lime, but nothing else and certainly no hard stuff. My first hangover was at Hendon Police College. It was my twentieth birthday and a true initiation.

My fellow rookies had taken me out and they'd bought me drink after drink. My poison was Pernod and black and they came thick and fast. I ended up pouring each one into a pint glass. By the end of the night I'd drunk two pints of the vile stuff. I went to bed very merry and very drunk, with a tongue that was warm, wet and black.

The next day I was ill. Very ill. Some joker suggested I drank milk, a 'great' hangover cure. Never having had a hangover before, I did as he suggested. The half-pint of cold semi-skimmed took less than a minute to come back up, curdled and purple. I was truly poisoned. There was no sympathy. To be unfit for duty through drink, or to be drunk on duty, are poor conduct matters that can lead to disciplinary action.

However, the trainers were forgiving as long as I sat in the classroom and did my work, didn't fall asleep and didn't puke.

It was a lesson that taught me quite early on about policemen and their drinking habits. I was a quick learner and I've never drunk Pernod since, but I didn't learn enough to stop me imbibing other poisons in the future . . .

It was customary for probationers to buy a round after their first arrest. And their first dead body. And their first court conviction. And every other opportunity that the 'old sweats' demanded. How we didn't end up bankrupt, I don't know.

Back then the shift used to mean working a whole week of night duty, then after finishing work on the Saturday morning, the guys would trot off to the Early House, a pub that opened at six in the morning for night-duty workers, post office workers, and those who worked in the markets like Smithfield and Spitalfields. The previous landlord of the pub had refused women entry, so female officers were exempt. However, a couple of years later he died and his son took over and for the first time the Early House saw women other than the regular Saturday-morning strippers. So of course when the doors opened, I had to go to the Early House. It was another obligatory initiation. Besides, the guys seemed to have so much fun on those Saturday mornings that I wanted to see what I was missing.

The first round cost me over twenty quid, which was a lot out of my spending money. The landlord took the opportunity those mornings to clean up his bar, so he only served pints and that was it. So I drank pints. Five of them . . .

Someone dropped me off home at my flat. I can't remember who. My parents were coming for a visit that night and as I was on nights they were going to stay over. I'd bought them tickets for the theatre. I don't remember them calling; my flatmate sorted them out. I woke up with less than two hours before I needed to be back at work for night duty. I was hungover and bleary-eyed and although very glad I wasn't a police driver, I didn't relish walking the beat in the cold rain. But, of course, it was obligatory.

Various stories that follow involve alcohol, and yes, you may assume that by the time I left the force I had been well and truly initiated. I could hold a drink or two. Or twenty. At my leaving do, I raised a glass of champagne and tried not to think of the innocent me of twenty years earlier, and how the alcohol-loving police officers got me in the end. Nor did I wish to remember the worst hangovers!

Cheers!

Prisoners, property and prostitutes

At training school we were warned about prisoners, property and prostitutes. If anything were to go wrong, it would usually have something to do with at least one of them. In the late seventies, around the *Life on Mars* years and before I joined the police force, I had dealings with all three.

Family circumstances had meant that I left home at seventeen and lived on my own in a cold and tiny flat opposite the sea. I needed two jobs to pay my bills, so I worked in an office during the week and in the cloakroom of a popular nightclub Thursday, Friday and Saturday. The money was rubbish but it helped. I fancied doing bar work, but the Fugly brothers who ran the tacky joint said I was too clumsy and not pretty enough. They may have had a point on the first and the book is open on the second.

One Thursday night, a long time after the supposed closing time, I was still at work in the club. It was about three in the morning and I was desperate to go home as I had to be up early for my office job. A drunken woman and her partner came to collect her coat but she couldn't find her ticket. She told me it was a white fur jacket with tissues in the pocket. There were three men's jackets and one white fur hanging on the rack. I found tissues in the pocket.

Maybe I shouldn't have given it to her but I did.

Half an hour later, the Fugly brothers tumbled down the stairs from their exclusive hidden bar, arm in arm with women I knew to be prostitutes, followed by half a dozen regulars – CID officers from the local nick, with their own cackle of voluptuous prostitutes.

The next night uniformed police came to arrest the elder Mr Fugly, a wiry ex-boxer, for knocking out forged fifty-pound notes. He was back an hour later, no charges and big fat grin. He sat at the corner of the bar, laughing.

'CID sorted me out. A case of mistaken identity,' he said, throwing back a slug of Scotch: Prisoners.

A few days later the brothers called me in to see them. The younger of the two had so many rolls of flesh around his neck that he looked as though he was wearing a scarf. With his bald bulldog head and flaccid bottom lip, he was intimidating. He stood over me, drool slavering down his chin as he ate a bacon roll. It made me feel sick.

Apparently, I'd given away the wrong fur jacket. The nightclub had secret CCTV cameras that nobody knew about, but I did now. It showed a woman handing over a ticket at 11 p.m. I gave her a fur jacket from the corresponding hanger. At 3.30 a.m. it showed me handing over the other fur jacket to the woman who didn't have her ticket. I could never understand how the first woman came by the ticket of a coat she says wasn't hers. Or how the second woman identified the remaining jacket, down to the tissues in the pocket. Yet they had the wrong coats. It caused mayhem and that was the end of my beautiful career in hospitality. Thanks to Property.

Many years later, I dealt with a case involving a family headed by a matriarch who openly declared that back in the day she'd been a prostitute who slept with policemen and gave them information. She knew one of the officers on the case.

'Old friends, sort of,' she said.

A short time later the officer took early retirement.

Aye. Prisoners, property and prostitutes.

In your face

After an enlightening time at Hendon I was posted to the heart of the East End. On the night of my passing-out parade I stayed with my parents at the pub they'd just taken over on the border of Essex and London. After the events of that night, I realised that night nothing in my life was ever going to be straightforward again.

Early in the evening my father ejected a drug addict for shooting up heroin in the toilets. The youth, Tony Atkinson, came back at midnight when the only people left were a small gathering celebrating my day.

The huge front window smashed into a thousand shards as Atkinson bounded through it, threatening us with a sawn-off shotgun.

My father didn't hesitate. He pulled back his old seafarer's arm and punched him once, knocking him to the floor.

I grabbed my virgin handcuffs from the bar where I'd been showing them off, and I jumped on top of Atkinson. I didn't think, didn't hesitate. Foolish really. Thankfully, he was out cold. I sat on his chest, grabbed his arms and snapped on the cuffs.

Technically he was my first arrest but I didn't go down on the custody sheet. The privilege went to the area car driver who was first on the scene. He was a decent arrest, what we called 'a good body' because Atkinson was wanted for offences of armed robbery, assault and drug dealing. The local police had been looking for him for weeks.

But the police didn't only arrest Atkinson. They arrested my dad, too.

Atkinson was conveyed to hospital with concussion, my dad to a police cell. I spent the night at the station giving a statement, defending my father against a potential charge of GBH.

Atkinson could have pressed charges against my dad, and threatened to do so. I didn't understand. No court would convict him, surely? It was a case of justified self-defence. Atkinson had a loaded gun and could have shot any of us. How was being knocked unconscious disproportionate to being threatened with and being in fear of a sawn-off?

It was a few weeks before we were informed there would be no further action taken against my father. Atkinson had done a deal and pleaded guilty.

It was certainly an introduction to policing.

A man's world

In the early days, they tested policewomen in a way they never would, or could, today. I resisted the arse-stamping initiation, something they did, or tried to do, to all new female officers and some civilian workers too. A swift tug of their skirts and down with the underwear, they'd try to brand their bottoms with the station stamp, a sort of 'you belong to us now'. I was very shy, embarrassed and could think of nothing worse. I wasn't going to let them get me, but they had me in other ways. Messages such as 'please ring Mr C Lion at London Zoo re an enquiry' or 'Mr Don Key at the local council'. One poor policeman was sent to the chemists to ask for some fallopian tubes. Like in many jobs, you learn to develop a sharp skill and quick wit that wasn't in the formal job description. I had a good right hook, should it be necessary. But they had me in other ways.

As the lone female probationer on a shift made up of men, I had to make the tea at the start of every shift and all the other breaks that policemen took. There was another woman on my relief but she was mainly on desk duty and she had much more service than me behind her, about four years more. Two guys started at the same time as me but they were *men*. It wasn't their job to make tea unless I wasn't there, then it was. However, I now make a mean cuppa, even if I can't stand the stuff, so I have to say thank you boys.

As in many predominantly male occupations, there was a lot of sexist behaviour. It's only now looking back that I realise the full extent. There was a lot of banter, some quite risqué, though I think there was general respect from most men and they didn't go too far. Many had wives, or girlfriends, or daughters and said they wouldn't want them to do the job, that it wasn't work for women. Older guys, those who'd done their time and were ready to retire, thought women should deal with the domestics, give out the death messages, look after abandoned or abused children and deal with sexual assaults. They remembered a time when there was a Police Woman's Department and female officers only dealt with those things.

When it came to the reporting of dead bodies, known as sudden deaths, the call was usually despatched to the probationers. It was down to them to deal with the families, the doctor, the undertaker, the paperwork and often attend the post-mortem (PM). It's an ideal way to get used to being a police officer and to learn how to be professional in such circumstances. It's the same today but back then, the priority went to WPCs. Make me or break me, malicious or mischievous, it was seen as toughening you up, and ultimately, you had to do it. Or get out. But times change and it's no longer like that. Yes, the first jobs probationers are given are still sudden deaths, shoplifters and civil disputes, but there are as many women officers as there are men, and sometimes more. Any hint of testing the metal in a sexist or racist or any other '-ist' way, and Professional Standards (previously known as Complaints) would come down and haunt you out of a job.

It might not have always been right, and some would argue there were quite a few wrongs in the way some people were treated back then, but we had a lot of fun and learned to laugh at ourselves as well as others. Earning respect and proving your worth is still good currency and I have no complaints about that.

But back then, I was given ten dead bodies to report on in my first five weeks and we used to have to attend the post-mortem for every sudden death we dealt with, unless it was a murder in which case it was a job for CID. By the time my probationary group had our official PM training session, I'd already been present at many.

Two of the men in my group fainted and one clung to a drain-pipe as he threw up in the swill yard (where the hearses delivered/ collected the bodies). I stayed long after we were dismissed to go home and discussed the procedure with the pathologist and the mortuary attendant, eager for information and willing to learn what I could.

I enjoyed my job – all of it, even if it did include a bit of death.

Face down in the gutter

My first dead body showed up on my second day on the streets. It was a cold, crisp early day in January and my tutor, PC Joe Gardiner, walked me along one of the busiest roads in the East End.

Traffic was building up. I took each step with trepidation, remembering the photo albums we'd seen at training school of fatal traffic accidents, murders and accidental deaths. We passed two of my fellow probationers stopping vehicles driving in the bus lane and I wished I could join them.

As we made our way up the main road I saw what looked like a bundle of rags up ahead by the kerbside. I felt giddy. This was it.

A few steps closer.

Another.

I saw it. Him. The body. A tramp. A dead person.

The world was going about its business, ignoring, or not seeing, the man frozen to the ground. PC Gardiner and I stood looking down at him.

'What are you waiting for?' Joe said.

I looked at Joe. Looked at the tramp. I felt the weight of my policewoman's hat on my head. I didn't know what to do, what to say. I was a fraud. I wasn't qualified to deal with dead bodies. I wanted to run.

I took a deep breath and crouched down, the hem of my skirt skimming the icy pavement. My stocking-clad legs were cold, as cold as the end of my nose and the tips of my toes in my polished black flat shoes, not yet scuffed by life. Or death.

I leant forward and could hear the sounds of traffic driving by, rattling engines and belching exhaust fumes. I looked at the man's face. Icy dewdrops had frozen on his white beard. He had frost in his eyebrows and on his eyelashes. A smattering of frosty spider web had settled in his dirty grey hair.

I pulled off my gloves and bent closer to feel for a pulse in his neck. I knew I wouldn't find one. There was something about his eyes. Glassy, non-seeing, half-open. The death stare.

He was a wizened old tramp with the stench of dirt and stale alcohol that wafted up my nose with my first smell of death. I touched the poor fibre of his clothing. Thin. So very cold. And old. Like his body. He might snap if we moved him. His face was white and purple and I wasn't sure whether it was bruising or lividity. He was half-curled, almost but not quite foetal.

'He's definitely dead,' I said.

'You the doctor now, Ash?' asked Joe.

'Hmm. No.' I thought about it. 'Do we call the doctor? Or do we need an ambulance?'

'An ambulance is for the living. Does he look like he's just died? Can we save him? You want to give him the kiss of life?'

I gulped, repulsed, embarrassed. 'No. No, I don't think so. But . . . I've never seen a dead body. How can I tell?'

Joe softened his tone. 'He's not warm. He's covered in frost. Okay, that could happen when he's asleep but there's no sign of life, no pulse and he looks like he's been here for some time.' He waved a gloved finger over the man's face. 'He's long dead.'

Joe called for the divisional surgeon, who wasn't a surgeon at all but a GP who was on call for the police and the only one who could officially pronounce life extinct. Each district had on-call doctors who worked on a rota basis and topped up their salary working for the police. Today they're known as Force Medical Examiners, or the FME. Ordinarily, we would call a deceased's own doctor, but we didn't know this man, or who his doctor was.

Scenes of Crime Officers (SOCO) only attended suspicious deaths or suicides, as would CID, so the rest was up to us, the uniform shift. I had to draw a sketch plan of where we'd found the body. I made a note of his clothing. We had to search the body and seize anything of value. In this case, there was nothing but small change. No wallet. No identification. Nothing.

Then we had to wait. And wait. And wait. The doctor came and pronounced life extinct, then the undertaker finally came to collect the body to transfer it to the mortuary. There was no point taking him to A&E.

Back at the station, PC Gardiner gave me the sudden death forms that needed completing for the coroner. My Girl Guide skills came in handy when one of the questions asked which direction the body faced. North-west.

'Fax it to the Coroner's Office,' Joe said. 'And be on standby for the post-mortem.'

Post-mortem. When I'd woken up that morning the last thing on my mind was a post-mortem. I hadn't thought about dead bodies. My head was full of chasing suspects, catching burglars, sorting out a lovers' tiff, my own romantic ideals. I'd never imagined I would be picking up a dead tramp by the side of the road.

Two o'clock that afternoon when I should have been clocking off duty, I stood by a metal trolley in the mortuary looking at the naked body of our unknown vagrant, the stench of death firmly entrenched in my nose and in my head. Today, I know that smell anywhere and can magic it up on a whim. You never forget.

The body of a very large man lay on the gurney next to our tramp. He'd been dragged beneath a bus for a hundred yards or more. Most of his skin was missing and the body looked black.

An old lady lay on the third trolley up. She'd had her post-mortem and her chest was stitched up in a 'y' shape. She was waiting to be put into the fridge before being taken to the undertaker.

If all of this shocked me, I wasn't prepared for the post-mortem itself. I didn't faint, I wasn't sick, but it was unlike anything I'd anticipated. It's not nice, not pleasant, but it *is* fascinating. And for the sake of the queasy, I'm not going to detail it.

Our tramp had frozen to death. Hypothermia. Such a sad way to die, lonely and cold and hungry. His last meal had been some chips about twelve hours before he'd been found.

I did cry a tear for him when our efforts to find out who he was failed. His fingerprints were not on the system and he wasn't known to police. He wasn't a regular vagrant around our area, so we sent a headshot to all the stations in central London. They failed to recognise him too, even though he'd obviously lived on the streets for some time. We checked and re-checked missing persons records to no avail. The local paper published his photograph and wrote an article about how he was found but still nobody came forward to claim him. Six months later, the council informed us he'd be given a pauper's funeral.

Who was he and where was his family? What had he done with his life? How and why had he ended up on the streets? When had he given up? Why? All of these questions remain unanswered. My first dead body: John Doe.

Nobody ever claimed him but I will always remember him.

Have you told her?

One of the most difficult and heart-rending jobs of a police officer is to tell someone a loved one has died. Like most jobs nobody wanted, the task of delivering a death message was given to the women or the rookies and for a time I was both. I was given them all. I hated it and often had to fight back tears as I gave the terrible news. I would rather have dealt with the actual death than have to inform the relatives. I'm the sort of person who cries at a stranger's funeral.

As soon as I came on duty one night, PC Jim McBean and I were sent to a house to pass on some bad news. We stood outside the door and I knocked twice. There was no answer but someone was at home because the television was flickering through the net curtains.

Jim rapped on the window.

A blonde woman pulled back the curtain. She was holding a crying baby and looked frazzled. She waved at us, indicating she would come to the door.

When she clicked off the latch and pulled the door open, my radio burst alive. 'Ash, have you told that woman her husband's dead?'

Not the way to deliver a death message.

Do not pass Go

If someone says don't look, you automatically get the urge to do just that, especially when it's a mangled car wreck.

There was a fatal accident at the bottom of a very busy junction, on the corner where a street market began. Shops and a pub and a betting shop lined the parade. One of those heavy super-armoured vans that are used to convey money had taken out a blue Volvo estate.

I was instructed to make sure nobody went past the police tape. After six hours, I was weary.

'But I live down there!' said an old man.

'Sorry. You'll have to wait,' I said.

'I only want to go a hundred yards,' said a man with a dog.

'Sorry. You'll have to wait.'

A woman with shopping bags approached. 'I have to collect something before the supermarket shuts.'

'Sorry. You'll have to wait.'

And so it carried on. I deflected all the pleas and fended off those who'd come to gawp. It was tricky as the van was laden with cash and it had to be gathered up and accounted for.

An irate woman approached and wouldn't accept that she wasn't going through. She was insistent, persistent and annoying.

My legs were aching, I was desperate for the loo, the forensic examination would be another few hours, and the PC assigned to take over from me hadn't turned up. I was grumpy and I wanted to go home.

'I don't care if you're the Queen of England, you ain't going down that road!' I rationalised it was human nature to lose it, all things considered. 'A man has been killed in that car this afternoon.'

She dropped her handbag and fell to the floor. She screamed and held her head in her hands and howled, oh how she howled.

I shouldn't have spoken to her like that. It was no excuse that I hadn't known it was her husband's car. I had just delivered the cruellest of death messages.

Gruesome twosome

They called us the Gruesome Twosome, my future husband and I. I suppose that's why we paired up. It put everyone else off. Whenever we were posted together, we ended up with a cartload of bodies, often the arrested kind but frequently the dead.

Kenny was one of those policemen who knew everyone and everything, with a mind like an encyclopaedia. Or the internet, had we had such a thing when I was a lass. He was a walking intelligence unit. People would ring him at home for a snippet of information because Kenny always knew everything about everything.

Kenny was married when I first met him. He was quite a few years older than me and far more mature. I was a young girl. A slip of a thing, as people used to say. He was attractive, I supposed, but I never looked at him in that way. There was never any suggestion of us getting together. He was happily married and I knew his wife. I always thought he'd make a great dad because he was so good with us probationers, as well as everyone else. He was the sort of policeman that you'd want with you when your back was up against it or you were knee deep in the cack. And he could talk his way out of most situations, too. People responded to him well. Perhaps it was that good old cockney way of his that he had honed to perfection. And I don't mean the likes of those you find on *EastEnders*. He was just an all-round good guy who treated people decently, whoever or whatever they were.

The first dead body we dealt with together was an old man, Mr George Chapman. He'd sat down in front of his television and died, his dog by his side. A neighbour who could see the man in his basement flat noticed he hadn't moved in between the hours of him going to work and coming back. The neighbour had a key but called the police before using it.

I was on foot patrol on my own and given the job. When I arrived, the neighbour let us into the flat. I naively said him, 'Have you seen a dead body before?

'I was in the war, love. I've seen my fair share, don't worry,' he said, with a wink.

I felt stupid but it was a lesson learned and although I'd already dealt with a few sudden deaths I was disconcerted to see Mr Chapman sitting there with his eyes half open, seeming to look at me wherever I moved in the room.

I called all the people I needed to call and I took a statement from the neighbour. Then I called for a unit to come and collect the dog. He'd have to go into kennels until we found the next of kin of Mr Chapman.

Kenny came to the rescue. He'd been posted to a panda and agreed to pick up the pet. 'Don't forget to search the house, Ash. Old people are notorious for stashing money away. The local burglars get wind he's died, they'll be in looking for it.'

I knew old folk did that because my granddad had done the same. Kenny left with the dog. I waited for the doctor and the undertaker to come and set about searching the bedroom, away from the half-open eyes. First stop, the bed. Cliché, yes, but there it was: a stash of fivers and ten-pound notes. I gulped. I collected it all up and looked in the bedside cabinet drawer. Apart from some loose change there was nothing of note. Then I looked in the wardrobe. It was one of those old-fashioned polished wood, curve-fronted pieces of furniture that were beautifully designed but out of favour. Just like the one my granddad had. On the shelf with the pile of old underwear was an envelope containing fivers. I checked the pockets of all the jackets and found more money. I called Kenny on the radio.

'When you've got a minute could you come back please?' I asked. 'And bring some property bags.'

'Aah,' he said. 'You've found what I was talking about then?'

'Umm. Just a bit.'

Kenny took it all in his stride. He checked the places I'd checked and then we searched some more. We counted it all up and it came to a few thousand quid.

'The neighbour who called it in can witness we've taken it. Any luck with next of kin?'

'I've got an address book. The neighbour said Mr Chapman had a couple of nieces who sometimes visit but he doesn't know where they live. I thought I'd ring some of the numbers in his book when I got back to the nick.'

'Good thinking,' said Kenny. He went off to get the neighbour while I transferred all the money to the kitchen table.

We counted £3,225, all in ten- and five-pound notes. We counted it twice. The neighbour acted as a witness and counted it with us. He signed our notebooks to agree it was correct.

On the way back to the station with the money all signed and sealed up, Kenny joked, 'They'll have to strip-search us you know. Check we haven't stolen any.'

I believed him. At first, anyway. He was a joker!

We booked it into Property and the station sergeant came to countersign it. He ripped open the seal and counted out the money. He counted it again. Then again. It was £100 short. What? How? I felt my insides go cold and I felt a little bit sick. I knew I hadn't taken any. I was confident Kenny hadn't either. I also doubted the neighbour had. So how?

Kenny checked the adding up on the original notebook entry. We'd written down a list of where each amount was found in the house. He totted up the totals again. The maths was wrong. In adding it up, somehow we'd included an extra hundred. The mistake was there to see.

We had to take the money and the notebook back to the neighbour. He laughed and said, 'It's all right. I know youse hadn't nicked any. I saw you make the mistake but thought I'd got it wrong. That it was my maths. Never my strong point.' He happily signed our notebook to that effect but I still worried about being questioned and strip-searched.

The next sudden death for me and Kenny took place on a cold and frosty Sunday morning in February. The puddles were iced over and the meagre day had only just begun. With not much else to do at six thirty on a Sabbath morning, we took a walk through an ancient cemetery.

I saw him first. He was sitting on a bench, slouched over a pair of old walking sticks. I suggested we took the other path, to allow the man some privacy.

'I think we'd better check him out. He looks a bit too cold to me,' said Kenny.

We approached the figure. Kenny touched the man's neck. He looked at me and shook his head.

I glanced down and on the path, between the man's legs, was a pool of congealed blood with a razor blade lying in it. Beside the man, on the bench, lay an unsigned letter.

It revealed his story. He'd visited his wife's grave and taken a seat on the bench. He had cancer and early dementia. He could no longer go on without his wife. He missed her so much. He was lonely. They didn't have children. He was an old man on his own and it was time to be with her again.

It was so very sad. I stood in the churchyard and cried. I wasn't tough. Not then.

Kenny was sympathetic and we dealt with the situation appropriately and respectfully.

A few weeks later, there was the man Kenny had to drag out of the river. I had to deliver the terrible news to the dead man's family when they came to the station to report him missing.

We had an old lady who had been dead in her bed for a week.

Then the young mum who had an undiagnosed heart complaint.

And there are many others we remember . . . lest we forget.

Hard-knock life

When that female chief inspector told us on our first day at training school that many of us would be injured on duty, I remember my throat constricting and my head giving a little wobble. I was clumsy and knew I could do myself an injury on my own without any help from anyone or anywhere else. I didn't like violence. I hated confrontation. Was I sure I was in the right job?

Yes. I loved it. All of it. Even when it was bad.

Black and white

I've policed many football matches when the Premier League was known as the First Division, and policed various marches and demos, but none so scary as my first, the Wapping dispute in 1986.

Two of the important roles of a police officer are to protect life and protect property. Whenever there are large demonstrations, marches and protests, it's everybody to the helm. Days off are cancelled, operational tasks rearranged, and whatever his or her regular posting, every officer needs to have a uniform ready for when duty calls.

The blistering, bubbling air was heady, heavy, as the capital prepared. In the bitter night, London waited. The festering pit of strikers, policemen and rubberneckers were gathering and sharp cracks of anticipation were interspersed with tingles of fear. The normally quiet streets of east London were like a boil about to burst.

Tired green battle-buses trawled through the streets as tetchy crowds swarmed on both sides of the metal barriers guarding News International. The cavalry arrived on glossy-coated beasts, many hands high and emblazoned with Metropolitan Police regalia. They incited fervour as they stomped and snorted excitement and fear, while their lord-like riders tried to still the rearing hooves. Fresh manure permeated the air, filling flared nostrils. Discordant horns and hooters joined the cacophony: sounds and smells of conflict.

Quiet chat grew to a low chant: '*Pigs, Pigs, Pigs, Pigs, Pigs, Pigs.*'

Keeping up the rear, dog-handlers struggled to keep anxious Alsatians in the back of their battered vans until the order for release came. It would, without doubt, come soon. Every animal instinctively sensed distress and unrest. Scurrying rats had long deserted their familiar streets and riotous disturbance chased foxes from urban undergrowth. Howls echoed in the night, as Man became Beast.

Like the last night of carnival, alive and electrifying, agitated tension filled the air as both sides prepared, the big wheel of misfortune turning. Hook-a-duck; hook-a-pig.

Politics had become lost, had nothing to do with the violence that converted convoluted words into an excuse for those wanting, waiting to fight. Genuine strikers, honest police officers and hearty politicians had no place in Wapping on 15 February 1986.

I was but a girl, naive and inexperienced, wearing a uniform tunic and skirt of heavy serge, with thin tights clinging to my legs because there were no trousers for women officers. Not then. My meagre arsenal comprised a handbag, a whistle and a little wooden truncheon, far smaller than those issued to the policemen. My new hard bowler hat had recently replaced the soft black and white peaked caps and I was thankful for that, at least.

Mike Bruce, my sergeant, must have seen my anxiety.

'We're the enemy, whether we like it or not. It's nothing personal,' he said, squeezing my hand. 'It was like this up the mines. Just stay close to me, Ash.'

I knew all about the mines. I'd lived in a town bordered by a dozen working pits. In 1984 I'd given 10 per cent of my factory wage to the families of the strikers because that's what those who were fortunate enough to be working did. The poverty of the proud pitmen, the despair of their conscientious wives, their children's hungry faces – they flashed back as the baying crowd chanted venom into my face.

'*Pigs, Pigs, Pigs, Pigs, Pigs, Pigs.*'

'But I'm not their enemy,' I whispered, fear catching at the back of my throat.

A duty, a job. To serve Queen and Country. I naively never expected to become an object of ridicule, to face such hatred. I only wanted to help people.

'*Oink, oink, oink. Pigs, pigs, pigs.*'

Someone shouted, 'Spit-roast porky-pig!' and the baying crowd jeered and hollered, thumping the air with lascivious encouragement. A kazoo sounded and a mounted officer danced his skittering horse to the back of the police barricade.

I looked around and saw two other policewomen. That made three of us in a crowd of 400 or more officers. Perhaps there were more hidden in the melee but I couldn't see them.

Wide-eyed and bewildered, I asked my sergeant, 'Why do they hate us so much?'

'We represent authority. We're the link between them and the powers in charge.'

'I know that. I'm not without sympathy. I understand. But it's not our fault.'

'Don't matter; they can't get at Maggie Thatcher so we're the next best thing. We're as bad as she is . . . to them. Maggie's boot-boys. Whether we personally support her or not.'

The atmosphere worsened as the crowds swelled, people pressing against steel barriers that were weakening at the surge of protestors and police officers.

'*Pigs, pigs, pigs, pigs, pigs, pigs.*'

'Keep your head down when the shit starts flying. Link arms and stay linked,' Sergeant Bruce shouted above the horde.

The inspector approached, tall and stern, yellow flak jacket standing out against the sea of bodies.

'They're out for it tonight, copper's blood. Remember Tottenham. Look out . . . and good luck.' He moved on, passing the unwelcome news along the line. Tottenham. It was only four months earlier that PC Keith Blakelock had been killed. He was at the forefront of every officer's mind. Barriers rattled, straining at the bit. A firecracker split the air. Cheering resounded in the inky night. Another battle-bus arrived, spilling open another packet of policemen tooled-up in riot gear. A heave forward pressed Sargeant Bruce and I against the metal barriers like we were cattle waiting to be herded into a truck. I was very afraid of being trampled.

A hand flew out, grabbing my hat. Someone pulled me backwards as the Velcro straps beneath my chin ripped open like weak packing tape. I clamped my hand down onto my hat and managed to keep on the only protective cover I had. Mike flung me behind him.

A sparkle of colour lit the night, showering reds and greens in shooting umbrellas of light that extinguished before they could settle on the restless mob. Cordite hung in the air as the fireworks intensified. Loud pops fired like showground rifles. Bangers whizzed and wailed, falling out of the sky and smattering into the crowd. Rockets speared the atmosphere like a dare. The taste of hatred, thick like treacle, clung to the insides of my mouth. Sour. Bitter. There was nothing sweet about this initiation.

Another yellow-coated inspector wound his way into our crowd, jostled among sweating police officers chomping and stamping, every creature farting and belching fear.

'Gold Command has ordered reinforcements. Rent-a-mob are expected to turn up. Most of the bloody force is out here tonight. Essex and Kent are on standby.

'Get her to the back of the crowd, Mike, it's no place for a woman.' He thumbed in my direction and moved on, spreading ill cheer.

'*OOO, OOO, OOO, oggie, oggie, oggie.*'

'*Pigs, pigs, pigs.*'

'*Lesbo, lesbo, lesbo.*'

Horns, hooters and whistles blew as fireworks continued to shoot. Nails, stones and broken bricks began to fly through the night; a maelstrom of powerful tools mingling with offensive diatribes. Police officers pushed from the rear as the shields, horses and dogs made their way to the front.

'Okay, Ash, when the shields get here, we'll move back,' Mike shouted.

'Right, sarge.' I had no intention of moving without him.

'*Pigs, pigs, pigs, pigs, pigs, pigs.*'

'*I'm forever blowing bubbles, pretty bubbles in the air . . .*' struck up a chord from the back of the mob.

'*OOO, OOO, OOO, oggie, oggie, oggie.*'

Heat emanated from both sides of the fence. Adrenalin flowed as sardine-packed policemen and strikers filled the streets. A police horse forged a way to the front of the crowd and I felt the animal's terror. I watched beads of fear roll down the smooth chestnut body of the beast, spittle flying from its mouth as his rider reined him in. The overpowering smell of leather, manure and hatred clung to me.

'*OOO, OOO, OOO.*'

The opposing team swelled by a few hundred more and the West Ham signature tune built to a crescendo.

The first petrol bomb fell wide and flames rendered the air orange with licks of fire.

'*OOO, OOO, OOO, oggie, oggie, oggie.*'

'Heads down!' a voice behind me ordered.

Our team crouched on command as another milk-bottle bomb flew our way. It landed at the forelegs of the stallion. He reared up, grand and foreboding, huge hooves turning as he spun. The metal arch of the horseshoe glinted as the rider was flung to the side, his foot caught in the saddle.

I skidded on fresh manure and rolled into the officer to my right as a hoof skimmed my left shoulder. The beast's other leg smashed down beside Mike. The poor horse fell onto his forelegs. I saw that the mounted officer had been pulled free from the horse by some officers and was being passed along the crowd like a hot potato, out of reach of the grabbing hands on the other side of the fence. Too hot to handle, he was jostled up into the air and thrown again and again into the back of our crowd.

The battle raged as Mike and I were carried out among the wounded, statistics from the strike. Eight officers were seriously injured, many more hurt. Fifty-eight arrests. Genuine protestors and police officers feeling the pain. Everyone scarred.

Twenty-five years later and 300 miles away, I watch on my television as a fire extinguisher is dropped from a great height onto waiting officers dressed in yellow jackets and black trousers, busy bees scattered across the foyer of a government building. A youth climbs a flagpole and defaces the Union Jack. Hundreds of students gather and protest against the proposed rise in university fees.

People complain about police tactics of kettling the crowd. A posse of schoolgirls guards a police van to stop vandals from ripping off doors and smashing windows.

Some months later a man is shot dead by police. There are lots of questions to answer. Lots of people angry. Rioters who have no idea why they are rioting take to the streets and loot and maim. Senseless violence. Many innocent people hurt.

I'm compelled to watch; I can't turn it off and can't turn it over. I'm there. On the streets. Fighting again.

I watch the scenes unfold from the comfort of home. I watch, remembering Wapping; the Poll Tax riots of 1990; the BNP march of 1993. And many others. Nothing is simple, nothing black and white. It might have been many years ago but nothing changes. There are always the police to blame.

Strapped

My first injury of significance was eight months into my probation. By the time it happened, I'd dealt with plenty of abusive, drunk and violent prisoners and I suppose I'd been lulled into a sense of security. When tackling someone who doesn't want to be arrested, or someone who wants to fight, you rely on your wits, your colleagues and your senses, one or all of which are prone to letting you down.

Female officers were armed with a little wooden stick, a truncheon, that was usually used to smash the windows of houses to which we needed to gain entry because the occupants were either avoiding us, or dead. We didn't have CS spray, or utility belts with heavy equipment to weigh us down. Nor did we have body armour. All that came later. Women didn't even wear trousers, mounted branch excepted.

It was a Friday night duty and I was posted with PC Jim McBean. I liked him. We got on well. He was a family man with four years' service and eight years older than me. He knew everything, everyone, and was what was known as an 'old sweat'.

It was nearing one o'clock in the morning, our refreshment time, and all the pubs had shut, or were closed having a landlord's private party, common practice in the East End on a weekend night.

Jim drove slowly past a block of flats on a notorious estate and I glanced into the car park as we passed by. I saw a stationary vehicle facing towards us, blocking the car park entrance. The headlights flicked off as we drove by.

'Can you go back, Jim? There's a car there. I don't know if it's stalled, or something. Maybe it's nothing,' I said.

Jim stopped and reversed back a few yards, pulling up in front of the car park. It was dark with the shadows of the building blocking natural light. The security lamp that was supposed to be lit had been smashed. We got out of the panda car and walked across to the purple Porsche. I heard the engine of the car ticking, cooling down. The driver's door creaked open and a tall dark-skinned man climbed from the driver's seat.

Jim called for a PNC check on the vehicle to see if it was reported lost or stolen and to find out who the registered keeper was.

The guy backed away into the car park, towards a stairway.

'Wait!' I shouted, rushing to the driver's door, which he'd left open. The ignition barrel was missing. The car had been hot-wired.

I ran to the stairwell and blocked the suspect from going into the building. He was broad and well over six foot and I felt tiny as he looked down at me. He did that sucking spittle in between his teeth thing.

'It ain't what you think,' he said.

Jim stood behind him.

The guy turned, waving his arms up in the air, as if brushing us away even though we hadn't touched him. 'You only stopped me 'cos I's black.'

'Rubbish,' I said. 'We stopped you because we thought there was a problem with the car. That you'd broken down or something. Whose car is it?'

He sucked into his teeth again. 'My mate's, man. I jus' stalled it.'

'You'll have the key then?' Jim asked.

I saw the man's head coming towards me but I couldn't do anything, go anywhere, my back against the stairs. He moved fast and smashed his head down onto my shoulder. The pain was like a metal spear shooting down through my chest. I fell to the ground. I know I screamed because I heard it, but it didn't sound like me. It was a yowling, yelping animal. The pain was sharp, sheer and I'd felt nothing like it before.

Jim grabbed him by his T-shirt, flung him up and then down in one sweeping motion in a swift black-belt judo move. The guy's head impacted with the tarmac and his left eyebrow split open. Jim pulled the prisoner's arms up his back and straddled him. I crawled towards them and hurled myself onto my attacker's legs, tights all tattered, my arm hanging limply.

Jim radioed for urgent assistance. When the cavalry arrived, the man, who gave his name as Colin Abehu, was taken away in the back of a police van. I was carted off to hospital for my shoulder to be set and strapped. It was dislocated and the collarbone smashed.

Abehu had a split eyelid.

The Porsche had been stolen from a financier who lived on the Isle of Dogs. Abehu was charged with theft of a motor vehicle and assault on the police. He admitted nothing and the case went to trial.

The jury found him not guilty on all charges. It was my first time giving evidence at Crown Court. I don't know why they didn't find him guilty. It left me with a bitter taste and a deformed collarbone and I didn't like it at all.

Knee-capped

My next injury was purely down to me being clumsy. I had to make some enquiries in relation to a credit card fraud and PC 'Garry' Garraway said he'd give me a lift. Garry was his nickname because police officers are nothing if not unoriginal when it comes to nicknames.

Garry manoeuvred the panda car into a small gap between a row of parked vehicles on Majesty Lane.

'Cheers, Gazza, I'll be about an hour, okay?'

'Yeah, just give us a call on the radio if I'm not here. I shouldn't be that long.'

I climbed out of the car and slammed the door. I turned towards the pavement. There was a good eight-inch gap between the bonnet of the panda car and the rear of the car parked in front of it. I didn't look. I didn't see. I strode on. I didn't account for the tow bar. Smack! The hard ball of iron slammed straight into my left kneecap. Another sheer ice-sharp pain that I remember along with the scream. I clutched my stomach to stop myself being sick over the police car. In an instant, my knee swelled to three times the normal size.

Garry shook his head as he helped me back into the vehicle. 'How long have you been back at work, Ash?' he said.

'Six weeks,' I grimaced.

That was the first time I dislocated my left knee.

Fitness test

I've always hated running. When I joined the force I managed to run a mile and a half in twelve minutes. Women recruits had to do it in a maximum of thirteen minutes, thirty seconds so I was pleased. But I still hated it.

These days police officers have to run after suspects while laden down with body armour, utility belts, handcuffs, radios, paperwork, CS spray, ASP (extending baton) and other heavy miscellany, so I suppose I should have been grateful I only had a truncheon, handcuffs, radio and a force issue handbag. In plain clothes it was a warrant card, handcuffs and if lucky, a radio.

I couldn't do it now, I'm not fit at all, but when I was, I caught many of those I chased. But there's always some you can't catch.

It was a frosty morning about 4 a.m. when a 999 call came out about a suspect being disturbed burgling an empty house. We ended up chasing a guy through a row of enclosed back gardens. Then we arrived at a six-foot wall. My male colleagues legged it up and over with aplomb. I jumped up on top – and stayed there. The drop on the other side was more than eight foot. I was stuck. I couldn't move because my skirt was hitched up thigh high, exposing my stocking tops and hindering me. To move I'd have had to pull my skirt up higher and slide one way or the other. It would never have happened if we'd had trousers.

I watched the guys bobbing up and over fences and walls. A gutsy yelp told me they'd caught their man. I sat and pondered my fate, hoping I wouldn't have to call for help. It was cold and painful and what if I ended up frozen there, on top of someone's wall?

I had to make a decision. Could I drop down one side? Could I get out of either garden without disturbing the occupants of the house? I couldn't see clearly as it was dark and I didn't have my torch because someone had borrowed it and forgotten to put it back. Or nicked it.

I decided to go for the longer drop because although the garden was derelict, I could see a path at the side of the house that might lead onto the street. I flung my handbag down first and, cursing, I pulled my skirt up to waist level. I leant forward and gripped onto the wall, then swung my left leg round to the right. My beautifully polished toecaps scraped the bricks at the same time as the inside of my thigh grazed the top of the frost-embossed wall. Ungainly. Unpleasant. Painful. I swung round and hung by both arms. I closed my eyes and dropped down, hoping I would manage to slide down the wall and miss the prickly bushes.

I managed but I snagged my stockings and gashed both knees. I felt around the cold earth for my handbag, snatched it up and clasped my sore palms together. If only my gloves hadn't gone missing. I admit my eyes were stinging a little as I tried not to feel sorry for myself and hobbled through the overgrown garden to the path that led to the front of the house. Hurrah! I was on the street. At least nobody had seen me.

The station wasn't far, so I walked back instead of calling for a lift. I knew they'd be busy with the prisoner. I sneaked into the toilets, tended my bloody knees and the stinging rash on the inside of my thigh, and bemoaned the damage to my shoes. I'd spent ages bulling them up. Tired and emotional, I wept. So much for being a rufty-tufty policewoman.

I cleaned myself up and went to the locker room where I changed my stockings and ran a black polish wipe over my shoes. It would have to do until I got home. I walked into the front office and Sergeant Matthews was by my side.

'There you are, Ash! Where've you been? We've been wondering what happened to you.'

'They nicked the burglar and I was way behind them so I walked back to the nick, sarge. I've been in the loo.'

'Why didn't you answer your radio? They're all out looking for you.'

'I never heard anyone call me,' I said. When I thought about it, I hadn't heard anything over the radio for ages. I looked down and it wasn't on. It must have been knocked off when I climbed down the wall.

'We had a 999 from a concerned woman. She said someone was sitting on her wall and she thought it was a police officer. A female officer.' He looked at me, eyes raised.

I looked back, eyes wide, lips schtum.

'Ash?'

'Well, I'm here, sarge. Might as well call the troops back,' I said.

I saw him look at my shoes. Then at my skirt covered in grubby brick dust.

I turned my back and mooched around my in-tray, hoping he wouldn't press it further.

He didn't.

He called the lads to tell them I was in the station and the caller must have been confused, a bit of night-time eyes.

In true back-covering protective fashion, he never mentioned it again. And neither did I, until today.

On prescription

I was minding my own business as I walked past Mile End tube station on my way to a briefing for a plain-clothes task I was involved in when a call came out that an intruder alarm had gone off at the chemist's. I was directly outside. I knew there had been three false calls at the pharmacy recently because they'd had a new system installed and staff had accidentally pressed the button. I also knew how busy it was at work, with people off sick, on leave and in court, so rather than tie up a patrol car, and even though I was in plain clothes, I said I would see what the problem was, fully expecting it to be another false alarm.

I was wrong.

I entered the shop and it was empty but for an assistant, a pretty Asian girl. She was crying.

'What's wrong?' I asked her.

'You have to leave, quick, the police are coming,' she whispered.

I showed her my warrant card and said, 'I am the police, what's up?'

'Are you on your own?' she whispered as she pointed to the back of the shop. 'He's in there with Mr Simon, the chemist. He's got a knife.'

I looked through the open hatch into the small back store.

Every shelf was packed with boxes and tubes and medicines teetering on top of each other. I saw Mr Simon standing in the corner and a tall man facing him with his back to me. The man had something in his hand but I couldn't see what.

I turned to the assistant. 'What's your name?'

'Maia,' she sobbed. 'He's after drugs. He's called Robert something and he comes in every day. He's on a script.'

'Maia, please call 999.'

'I can't. The phone's out the back. That's why I pressed the alarm button.'

I handed her my radio. 'Go out onto the street and use this. Press that button and tell them who you are and what's going on. Tell them an officer is here and I'm on my own and that the man has a knife.'

She took my radio, sniffled a bit and nodded.

I went behind the counter and picked up a foot aerosol, the only thing I could think of to arm myself with as I walked into the medicine store.

'Hello?' I said.

The man turned, thrusting a large knife. It was a horrible-looking thing that flashed silver in the sharp strip light, six or seven inches with a serrated edge.

'Get out!' he roared at me.

'I'm a police officer. I'm on my own. Please put the knife down.'

'I want the drugs in his cabinet. I know where he keeps them. It's locked. If he gives them to me you can both go. Right? Right?'

Mr Simon shook his head. The room was strangely silent, no sounds from outside at all; it was like being cocooned in an egg box.

'I'll tell you one more time, open the cabinet,' Robert said sweating, his pupils tiny pinpricks, his face a waxy pallor with a look that matched the desperation in his voice.

I hoped the troops would arrive soon. I tried to reason with him. 'We'll talk about the drugs but you don't need the knife.'

The chemist stepped forward.

I shook my head at him and turned back to Robert. 'You really don't want to hold up a police officer, do you? It's only going to make things worse. Put the knife down. Do you have a regular script?'

'Yeah, yeah I do. But I need more and he won't give it to me.' He wiped his sweating forehead with the back of his hand. He was agitated.

'You don't look very well,' I said.

Time stood still. Nobody said anything; the air was tense, the mood sharp. No one wanted to make the first move.

He stepped towards Mr Simon. 'I need the drugs. Now. Just get me the drugs.'

The chemist said, 'Robert comes here every morning and I give him his prescription. He was late today and he didn't come yesterday and he missed a few days last week. I know he's been getting it from the chemist in Poplar. I wasn't going to give him it again.'

Robert swung the knife up towards Mr Simons' chin. 'Shut up. Shut up!'

I stepped forward at the same time as Mr Simon. We both bumped Robert and the knife clattered to the ground. I kicked it away and it slid beneath a cabinet. Between us we wrestled Robert, who was more than a bit uncoordinated, and we made him lie face down on the floor. Just at that moment half a dozen uniformed officers hurtled into the tiny room.

'What kept you, boys?' I said, my heart pounding in the well of my throat.

Robert Miscow came from a well-to-do family. He'd dropped out of university and got into drugs. He received a six-year prison sentence for armed robbery. Mr Simon and I received commendations. I can't help thinking it was all a bit mad, a bit sad and a bit dangerous.

And that's just what I loved about my work.

No headway

Unfortunately for him, PC Jim McBean was often posted with me. I say unfortunately not because I didn't work hard, or that I was difficult to work with, or that we didn't get on. We did. I say it because when we worked together, we attracted trouble.

Sergeant Flint posted us together one Sunday night duty. 'Keep out of mischief, you two. You know what I mean.'

Everyone laughed.

It was about two thirty in the morning when we were called to a domestic on the eighth floor of a tower block. We were the only unit able to attend as half the shift were on their meal break (usually known as 'refs' for refreshments), and those that had the earlier slot were busy dealing with prisoners.

As is the way when you are in a hurry, both lifts were out of order and so we had to take the stairs. After climbing sixteen flights of stairs in a rush, I was exhausted. I could hardly breathe, never mind speak.

There were four flats to each landing. The door to the one we were called to, number 803, was open. It led into a hallway that turned left, I presumed into another part of a hall with doors off it to the other rooms, including the sitting room. All was quiet, not a sound.

'Hello!' I shouted. 'It's the police.'

'Anyone home?' shouted Jim behind me.

Silence when you arrive at a domestic could mean a number of things. It might mean it was a false call. Or maybe one half of the domestic has left. Rarely, there might be a dead body, or even two. The mind runs wild for a moment and then calms down as you realise they've probably made up and gone to bed.

I turned to Jim, tutted and walked down the short hall. Before I had time to think, a man steamed around the corner at me, brandishing a bread knife in each hand. He lunged straight for me, screaming, 'Arrrrrggggggghhh!'

My instant reaction was to put both hands up in front of my face. I closed my eyes. I didn't immediately feel the pain. That came once I'd seen the blood. I fell to the floor, thick red covering my hands like gloves.

I was aware of Jim jumping over my head and tackling the man, throwing him to the ground in that good old judo way of his.

Two women came out of a room, huddled together, crying. One of them grabbed the knifeman's leg and bent it up as he and Jim lay in a bundle on the floor. I fought through the jumble of arms and legs and scrabbled for the knives.

Brian Petch was rabid, like a wild man, with a guttural screaming that seemed to come from his belly. He had super strength and it took everything Jim and I plus the two ladies had to keep hold of him. I can't remember which one of us called for urgent assistance but someone did. It seemed to take an age for anyone to arrive but then I remembered – the lifts weren't working.

When the cavalry did come, they came in droves. When the call goes out that an officer has been injured, everyone comes, from your district and beyond. Adrenalised comradeship, an innate desire to be there, to give assistance, to protect, and to apprehend. And indignation that a man is down.

Despite at least a dozen uniformed police officers and the two night-duty detectives, Petch still tried to make a run for it. He hadn't bargained on meeting the dog handler on the stairs.

Joey the police dog took a tasty bite of upper thigh for his supper. It meant a lot of work and report writing for his handler, but Joey was given extra biscuits and plenty of pats on the back for making the arrest.

I was lucky to escape with injuries to my hands only. I was patched up with stitches and bandages and went back to the station. The impact didn't hit me until I sat nursing a cup of hot sugary tea. It had happened so fast. The shock was as much about what could have happened as what actually did – how he could have stabbed me, how it might have ended – and the thoughts bounced around my head. I couldn't stop thinking about it and sat there shaking.

Petch was a drug addict who'd just been released from Pentonville prison. He hadn't had any drugs for months but had taken something that night which had had a strong effect on him. He'd turned up at the flat of the guy he'd been sharing a cell with, looking for a bed because his pal had promised he could get one there. He found the man's wife with a woman, her lover, and went berserk, even though it was nothing to do with him.

Petch was charged with GBH with intent to endanger life. It was before the days of the CPS (Crown Prosecution Service) and the case files had to go off to a department somewhere centrally for them to arrange representation by the force's legal branch. It used to be the police decision on prosecutions, guided by legal experts they employed, whereas the CPS are now independent. Is it better? Probably. It takes the onus away from the police and they can concentrate on investigating and not prosecuting, purely gathering the best evidence they can. For reasons I will never understand, perhaps saving costs or some other initiative of the time, the case was dropped from GBH to common assault. Common assaults in those days weren't prosecuted in the magistrates' court but referred to civil remedies which meant making a personal case at the civil court, a private prosecution between the two parties, rather than a public one paid for by the state.

We appealed but lost our fight.

To go out onto the streets to protect the public, to be stabbed by a raving knife-wielding maniac, only to be told it didn't really matter, that it was just a common assault, was a kick in the gut for all proactive police officers. My physical scars healed but I felt very let down.

An independent barrister read of the case in the *Police Review* magazine. He contacted me and asked if he could take my case on as a private prosecution because he felt strongly about this miscarriage of justice. He had successfully dealt with similar incidents involving police officers over the past year and he was happy to fund it through his firm, pro-bono.

I agreed.

The Metropolitan Police couldn't be seen to endorse this course of action, but every officer involved in the case backed me and agreed to be present at the hearing, as did the civilian witnesses, including the doctor who had treated me. I was anxious but positive.

Due to a certain amount of legal wrangling it took over a year for a final court date to be set. Exactly a week before the hearing was due to start, I received a phone call at home from Surrey Police. There had been an accident on the M23. Brian Petch was the front-seat passenger in a car being driven by another well-known criminal who was high on drugs. Petch had been decapitated.

There was more.

'Oh, I nearly forgot,' said the traffic officer. 'You'd better get yourself tested. Did you know he had AIDS?'

Moving west

I enjoyed my time in the East End and it was a great place for a policing apprenticeship. I had worked in uniform, done a six-month home-beat posting, worked in plain clothes and had a stint on a murder team, but it was time to move on.

When I first applied for an undercover posting, the interview panel was made up of a detective chief superintendent and a detective inspector. I was overawed and stuttered over my words as I tried to tell them about my aptitude for detective work. I told them how I'd single-handedly arrested a robber armed with a knife and about being stabbed. I mentioned the times I'd given evidence in Crown Court and how I'd dealt with copious dead bodies.

They asked questions I was able to answer both in theory and with practical examples. I don't know if I impressed them or not. It didn't work like that.

When I didn't get the posting my sergeant said, 'Never mind, Ash. You can always try again.'

I vowed I would, and in the meantime, I planned to work harder than ever, even if it did mean looking for other opportunities.

* * *

When the call came out for officers to go to central London, which covered the West End, I put myself forward. I was ambitious and loved a challenge. My ultimate goal was to work undercover, so as much experience as I could get would be invaluable.

I was twenty-three and the people I'd worked with during the previous four years were like a family. I'd moved from the section house accommodation above the police station and was now living in a flat further east, but still in the heart of a wonderful community.

I was sad to say goodbye but it turned out to be one of the best career moves I made.

All the evidence

Policing the West End is very different to policing the East End. You still deal with crime and life and death and the public, but the West End is full of tourists, people looking for entertainment and bright lights, as well as the people who live and work there.

I hadn't realised how many gaps I had in my education until I entered the Collator's office in my new nick. (These days the Collator is better known as the LIO, or Local Intelligence Officer.) I stared at the various mug shots labelled Van-Draggers, Clip Joints, Dippers, Rent Boys. Where were the TDA merchants (taking-and-driving-away – also known as twockers – taking without owner's consent), the robbers, the burglars?

It was enlightening to learn about these new-to-me crimes. Most of our suspects in the West End lived 'off the ground' rather than on it. They'd come and do their dirty business on our patch then wander off again, so we had a sea of transient faces to get to know and it was hard graft.

It wasn't long before I learned about a crime unique to areas like Soho.

Mark Stamper, a tall good-looking guy, stumbled down a busy Soho street with a tissue held to his mouth. He had blood on his hands and his suit jacket was ripped. He held the tissue away from his face to reveal a nasty cut on his lip. He said he'd been approached by a black guy in his thirties, meaty and six foot, with a short Afro, and wearing a black Puffa jacket. He said the guy produced a chisel and demanded his wallet.

'He threatened to stab me, officer,' he said.

'Did you give him your wallet?' I asked.

'It had my bankcard in it but no money. He grabbed my arm, ripping my jacket, and then he marched me to the cashpoint. He made me take out 500 quid, my limit,' Mr Stamper said, on the brink of crying. 'My wife will go mad.'

I noticed the cut of his suit, the quality shine to his shoes, and the smooth leather of the wallet he showed me. Something about his little tale didn't ring true and it was a script I was becoming familiar with.

'I see,' I said. 'Where were you before this man approached you?'

'Just a little place having a drink.' He didn't meet my eye. 'The guy head-butted me and stabbed me in the hand, officer. Will you take a statement?'

'Which little place?' I asked.

'It's not relevant, is it? I was walking along the street when he attacked me.' Mark Stamper became irritated, edgy, and there was a distinct lack of eye contact.

'We could go and retrace your steps, from this little place to where he stopped you . . .' I played his game but he decided he didn't want to play anymore.

'Forget it,' he snapped.

'Absolutely not. You've been assaulted. Robbed. Aggravated robbery is a serious offence.'

'I don't want to cause a fuss. Can't you just give me a crime number or something? I need to get home.'

'Would you like me to call your wife, Mr Stamper? Our control room can let her know you're all right.'

'No!' he shouted. 'No. No need for that. I don't want any trouble.'

I took Mark Stamper to the station and sat with him in an interview room off the front office. I gave him a cup of tea and took his statement, reminding him that in signing it he was making a true declaration. He decided he couldn't remember which 'little place' he'd been to as he wasn't familiar with Soho and he certainly wouldn't be coming back. The cashpoint was at the bottom of a busy street, near Regent Street. I knew which one it was and I told him it had had CCTV installed recently.

Mr Stamper then decided he didn't want to make a complaint after all.

I gave him my details and reminded him again that assault was serious and we would certainly like to deal with that, even if he changed his mind about the robbery.

I knew he knew that I knew. I also knew he wouldn't pursue it further.

It was a familiar story. These 'little clubs' – clip joints – smaller than a sitting room, advertised *Girls, Girls, Girls* who, for a fee, would sit with gentlemen and encourage them to buy drinks, drinks that were 2 per cent alcohol, not what it said on the bottle. They'd charge the guy £45 for half a glass of watered-down fizzy Pomagne, companion service included. When he made to leave, he'd be stung for a bill of £300, £400, £500 or more. The price included the 'company' of the short-skirted, usually stoned hostess who'd waggled her bikini-topped breasts into his face and stroked his trouser leg. When these men wouldn't, couldn't pay, they'd be frog-marched to the nearest cash machine to withdraw everything they had. Protestations were met with a threat, maybe a head-butt, and sometimes a jab or two. The money would be withdrawn and handed over. The majority of these men refused to tell the truth, ashamed, embarrassed and caught out having to admit they'd been in a girly club, so we'd receive an allegation of cashpoint robbery instead of the real version of events. Most of the victims had families and could ill afford fifty quid, never mind five hundred, so they reported it as a street robbery, a credible excuse to their partner to account for the missing money because there was no way they were going to tell the truth – that they'd been in a club with women of lower moral standards.

I don't know who they were trying to kid: us, their wives or themselves. It *was* robbery, and often menacing, and it did sometimes include assault, but the perpetrators got away with it because nobody wanted to say they'd gone to a clip joint. The thugs knew this and exploited the situation.

Sometimes, someone surprised us and told the truth. We'd then go back to the club and demand their money back. The door gorilla would produce the small print at the bottom of the sticky menus that listed the extortionate prices for company and for drinks. It then became a civil dispute because what these men hadn't realised was that by sitting down with a girl and ordering drinks, they'd agreed to the terms and conditions. If there had been an assault, we could arrest the attacker, but more often the victims refused to cooperate with police when they realised they'd have to give evidence in court.

On some occasions we'd carry out an operation to stop it, but there are always guys wanting to take a chance with a girl in a club and while there's demand, there will always be heavies who won't let them get away with it.

The night I met . . .

I'll never forget the night duty I was sent to Jermyn Street, W1, to stand by while filming was taking place. It was just another job in the day in the life of a young constable in the capital. There was always filming taking place somewhere in the West End. Most of it happened at night when the streets were quieter and there were less people around. It was a boring task but once in a while something exciting happened.

There I stood, scuffing the pavement while keeping the non-existent crowd at bay, and trying not to lean against the metal barriers, which were more for effect than protection. I was bored and dreaming about my warm bed, thick blankets and a deep sleep. I had no idea who was filming, what they were filming or when it would finish.

A distinctive voice crooned in my ear, caressing the air with a tone like velvet. 'Aren't you cold, my dear?'

I was startled and compelled to look up. I fell into pools of sparkling blue as his twinkling eyes smiled at me. Wow! This man oozed sex appeal even though he must have been thirty or more years older than me. Age didn't matter on this cold autumn night.

I smoothed down my skirt, coarse under my fingertips and

unbecoming as a fashion item for a young girl like me. 'Err . . . a bit . . . yes . . . chilly,' I stuttered.

He was much taller than I'd imagined.

'Don't they give you trousers these days?' he asked, eyes sparkling, mouth crinkling, everything about him charming and easy.

I smiled back. 'Not yet. Maybe in a couple of years, when they catch on.'

'In my dad's day,' he said, 'when he was a sergeant at Bow Street Police Station . . .'

And that's how I became star-struck for a man older than my father. I spent a very nice half an hour with this gorgeous man, alone in his company. He told me all about his father who policed like policemen should back in the wartime years. He told me about his childhood and what it was like to have a policeman father and how he was both in awe and just a little bit frightened of him. How they were given oranges and lumps of Christmas pudding in their stockings at Christmas and if they were lucky they'd get a sixpence. Or maybe half a crown.

He asked questions about me and appeared interested in the answers, things like why I'd gone to London, what my ambitions were and what did my family think. He said he hoped I'd live my dream, just like he was living his.

He might have been acting, or he might have meant it. I don't know. I was sorry when he had to go back to filming. Like a true fan, I was enamoured. I was also a smidge embarrassed when I asked for his autograph. I still have it, written on a piece of Metropolitan Police memo paper.

I'll never forget the night I spent half an hour with Roger Moore.

He was the first of the big stars I was to fall for . . .

Up the junction

To be authorised to drive a police car you have to pass a police-driving course. This meant six weeks of intensive training, at the end of which you had to pass a final test. This was far more advanced than a normal driving test. It was exhausting, hard work and rigorous, with a lot of theory to learn.

In the Metropolitan Police, the driving school is based at Hendon Police College, now known as the Peel Centre. Each course would have five or six teams of three officers posted with an instructor. We would work all day driving fast and strategically in unmarked cars through country lanes, in towns and on motorways. We had a day on the skid pan, which most of the guys loved, a day driving a double decker bus on an airfield, and a day changing tyres, fan belts and learning about other mechanical things.

I took great care and concentrated hard but it didn't come easy to me. My head spun every night of every day of the course. It didn't help that my instructor, Frank Parrot, wasn't a very nice man. He was a civilian trainer and fancied himself as a cop. He also had old-fashioned ideas and asked me why I wasn't at home looking after a husband and some children. He said he didn't understand a woman wanting to do a man's job.

'Unless you're one of those lesbos? Are you?' he asked me on the second day.

I didn't reply. He said many objectionable things. I didn't agree with his views, and he had many, but I kept my mouth shut. I wanted to pass the course.

One of the guys in my car, Laurie, was chatty, a bit of a wide-boy, which was okay because he kept the instructor talking and I didn't have to say much. The other guy was Rhys. He was Welsh, about my age, married and a bit quiet. He was lovely.

We were in the fifth week and it was a baking hot day. The rapeseed was vibrant yellow and the air pungent as we drove through the country lanes of Essex. My eyes were fuzzy and I thought I might have a touch of hay fever to add to the fatigue.

I'd driven about a mile when the instructor told me to put my foot down and drive faster. I was already doing sixty. I wasn't familiar with the roads and I wasn't that confident. He was encouraging me to do an overtake I didn't feel safe making. He prodded me in my ribs, sharp and hard.

I gasped.

'Are you an excessive overeater or just naturally fat?' he said.

'What? What?' I couldn't believe what he'd said. I tried to keep focus on the road. I was furious. How rude. How nasty. I wasn't even fat! My face burned bright red. The sun glared into my eyes as I drove around a blind bend, and I sneezed.

Up ahead I saw an indent in the road, a farmer's track or gateway. I pulled in and stopped the car. I got out and slammed the door. I didn't want to but couldn't help crying at this point. Hot tears spilled down my face. I'd had enough of being baited and bullied by him, pushing me to fail. I knew I would fail. He didn't like me and he'd make sure I didn't pass. He made no disguise of the fact he thought women couldn't drive. I knew I made silly mistakes and he made me nervous, which made it worse, but I wanted to pass so much. I needed to, not just for the station but for me, so that I could go into surveillance because you had to have the driving skills for that kind of work.

I could see the instructor laughing in the front passenger seat. Bastard!

Rhys got out of the car. 'He was out of order. I'll back you if you want to make a complaint,' he said.

I was heartened. 'Thank you. I don't know what I'm going to do but I'm not getting back in that driver's seat. Not with him.'

'It's okay, I'll drive.'

We stood a few minutes longer. Rhys climbed into the front seat and I took his place in the back. Frank said nothing and neither did we.

Once back on the motorway, Parrot looked at me through his rear-view mirror. 'Over your little tiff now?' he said.

I ignored him and looked out of the side window. I was still flushed, still furious, and determined never to drive with him again.

When we got back to the training school I gathered my things. I had to carefully consider my next move. I was young in service. I couldn't and didn't want to refuse to go back. My shift needed me to pass this course because we were short on drivers. And I wasn't a quitter.

I went back the following morning and asked to see Sergeant Thomas, the officer in charge. He was also an instructor and his team were getting ready to go out.

I told him what had happened the previous day and on other days during the previous five weeks. He listened, nodded, made sympathetic noises. I had the impression I wasn't the first person to complain about Mr Parrot.

Sergeant Thomas told me my instructor hadn't given me good weekly reports. He said he was surprised because he'd seen me driving on various days and thought I was doing okay. He was a man down in his car because one of his students had gone off sick with chicken pox so he said I could go with him.

I had the best drive ever. Sergeant Thomas said he was impressed and there was no reason why I should fail. Yes, I was a careful driver, but I didn't hesitate or hold back.

The next morning Sergeant Thomas took me to one side before setting off for the drive.

'Rhys came to see me last night. He's backed up what you said. You're in my car for the rest of the course and I'll be taking you for your test. You can make a formal complaint if you want to, Ash.'

I didn't want to do that. I couldn't because it would be difficult. I'd be branded a troublemaker, labelled as a grass, someone who couldn't take a joke. I'd been allowed to change instructors and was beginning to believe I could pass the course. If I complained it would mean internal discipline for Parrot. He would deny it and then what? Perhaps naively, I hoped this would be enough for him to not do it again. I didn't want to drag Rhys into it either. I had no idea what Laurie would say but I had a feeling he wouldn't want to get involved.

'I spoke to Frank Parrot,' Sergeant Thomas said.

My body slumped.

'He said he was putting you under stress, making you drive under pressure, because on the streets you have to be able to keep calm while driving fast police cars with the blues and twos on. You might have to deal with an urgent assistance, or a robbery in progress, or something high tension and he said he wasn't sure you could handle it.'

'Really? You really think that's what he was doing?' I said. 'He knows nothing about me or how I do my job. He's plain nasty. He was doing it because he could, because he thought he could get away with it. Is that how you teach your pupils, sarge?'

The sergeant shook his head. 'Err . . . no.'

Nothing more needed to be said. We both knew the truth of it.

I didn't make a formal complaint. Today, I probably would, but I'm older, wiser and less intimidated. Back then, I was just grateful to pass the course. And I did. One up to me and one down to Parrot. I guess I was triumphant because it wasn't just about passing the course: it was a turning point. Sometimes you have to fight to realise that nobody has the right to make you feel like that but they will if you let them. It was good for my confidence to win that round and move on.

I wasn't the first and I wasn't the worst affected. Lots of women, and some men, had it harder, harsher and it wasn't fair. Thankfully the police service has come many miles since those days.

Bounty hunting

After a couple of years working in the heart of London, I was beginning to think it was time to move on. I loved it very much but six years into my career, with experience of two very busy districts, it was time for the next challenge. It was almost Christmas and each day was hectic with shoppers, partygoers and tourists, with an added dash of criminals looking for rich pickings. It was a great place to work with a vibrant atmosphere, sparkling Christmas lights and the ambience of good will to all men. It would be a shame to leave my uniformed colleagues but uniform street patrol wasn't something I wanted to do forever. I didn't have time to think too deeply but having made the decision, I decided to see what the New Year would bring in 1992. January was always a good time for change.

With three and half days left of the year, the prisoner count stood at 9,800. The superintendent returned to work after his jolly Christmas break in festive spirits and good humour. He laid down a challenge. The person who brought in the ten thousandth prisoner of the year would receive a decent bottle of Scotch. He was confident that 200 prisoners wouldn't pass through the doors between then and the chimes of Big Ben bringing in New Year.

Everyone wanted that bottle. How far it would go on a shift of perhaps twenty or thirty officers, or an office full of CID detectives, was a moot point, but it was a sharp tactic to get everyone working over the usual lull between the festive bank holidays.

CID scoured the crime books for outstanding arrests and warrants. Street Crime Units were extra vigilant in arresting street entertainers, those selling knock off perfume and other goods on the crowded pavements, plus the prostitutes and rent boys. The crime squads worked hard at the pickpockets and van-draggers (people who steal from the back of delivery vans) and drug dealers. Each uniform shift cleaned up Soho, arresting vagrants and druggies, and fought over calls for shoplifters, breach of the peace and other miscellaneous fights and disturbances. A three-day initiative on drink driving was implemented around Mayfair and St James. More cars than usual were pulled up for minor offences because you never knew when a regular stop would lead to something more. Between now and the end of the year everyone was working hard. Instead of warnings and cautions and let-offs, we operated a zero-tolerance approach.

You could say the period between Christmas and New Year that year was one of the most productive ever recorded in the West End. The prisoner count crept up. By the time my shift came on night duty on 29 December it was 9,852.

There was no way we'd be able to arrest more than a dozen miscreants between us because there were only six of us on the streets that night. With the usual calls to deal with, unless there was a big incident, even a dozen would be pushing it.

When we came back on duty the following night, the station had been busy and the count stood at 9,966. We knew the early-turn relief would nab that bottle if we didn't, so in our parade briefing we devised a plan of action. We needed thirty-four prisoners booked into custody. We had ten officers on duty. The area car was double crewed and could deal with the 999 calls and anything else they could fit in. The two vans could lose their escort, which gave us six-foot soldiers. We prayed nothing major was going to happen. If it did, we'd be done for, and and those bandits on the other shifts would get the booty.

Come mid-shift the world would have settled down and that's when our plan would kick in.

By 2 a.m. we were up to 9,972. Everyone agreed to forfeit their refreshment breaks and get back out there until we were done.

The drunks, vagrants, beggars and other assorted street people were rounded up and brought into the station in the back of the van, six at a time. We each took a prisoner, booked them into custody, gave them a caution, and released them back onto the streets, only to be found loitering or drunk again. Then the next six were brought in, processed and chucked out. Word soon travelled the itinerant community and we even had a couple of youngsters turn up at the front desk asking if they could help out and be arrested because it was ever so cold out there and they could do with a warm place to stay.

We obliged a sleeping vagrant who was particularly grumpy about being woken up in his comfy doorway. We agreed to give Wilf a bed for the night and breakfast in the morning in return for his cooperation. Everyone was happy.

Poor Archie Meehan, riddled with lice and addled with alcohol, was given three cautions that night, but he embraced it. He wanted to be the 10,000th prisoner and we gave him the privilege at 5.30 a.m. He raised his arm and said he was going down in history. It was one of his proudest moments, he said. I'm sure someone must have slipped him his favourite tipple as a reward.

Of course, rumours reigned about who the arresting officer was. I was never sure, not exactly, and I can't lay claim to it being myself, but I was there and took my part along with the best of them.

It was never about the bottle of Scotch. It was about other things altogether. It was one of the best of times and that night the street people did us proud. In the true spirit of working together, it was sublime. And a great way to round up the year.

Nondescript

I'd always wanted to work in plain clothes, to do detective work, to investigate crime. Perhaps it was too many Enid Blyton books as a child and too many detective novels growing up, but the idea of covert surveillance fascinated me.

I did a short secondment on an elite team, the crème de la crème of undercover units. The girl did good. I learned new techniques, discovered many methods of surveillance, more than I knew existed, and how to read street maps upside down. I thoroughly enjoyed it. I received a recommendation and a heads-up when the next vacancies came around.

Craig Baker, the sergeant in charge of the undercover unit, said that I would do. I was good for surveillance. They needed more women on his team and I was perfect, nondescript, unmemorable, perhaps a tad too tall but I could mingle in a crowd, blend into a sea of faces without encouraging a second glance.

Charming. I didn't know whether to be pleased or insulted but it didn't matter. I got the job.

Wheel clampers notorious

When you're due to move stations or into another role, you ideally clear up your current and outstanding cases. You also need to keep out of trouble. It's not unusual to be posted as station officer, or gaoler, or be given some other inside position during the weeks before you move on.

I was due to go off and work incognito, so the sergeant posted me to the clamp van. I hated working the clamp van. If you want to go to Traffic or had an interest in motors, then it might be a good posting, but for those like me who preferred dealing with crime and with people, it was loathsome.

As a probationer I did my quota of traffic offences. I reported people for driving in a bus lane, for doing red lights (which I agree is very wrong), for parking on a zebra crossing and for driving a car in a dangerous condition. I did what I had to do as directed by my performance indicators. Once out of my probation, if I presented my sergeant with a traffic process book, once he had picked himself up off the floor, he knew the offence must have been something bad.

Speed kills, yes it does, but I much prefer nicking those involved with a different kind of speed. Therefore, to be posted to the clamp van was my worst nightmare. Not only did it mean getting to work for 9 a.m. and travelling during rush hour, but it also meant I'd have to upset at least thirty people a day, which I hated doing. And I went home smelling of man-van, metal and oil.

The local council ran the clamping department. It had been agreed at a high level that each clamp van should be manned by a trained clamp person (a clamper) and a police officer who had to write the tickets. I can't remember exactly how much it cost the driver to have the clamp removed but the total cost of ticket and clamp was very expensive. The clampers were council workers not trained in people skills. Nor did they have the vetting police officers had. Some of them were great guys (there were no women clampers) but others were like bulldogs, or gorillas. Neanderthals. And I had a thirty-day posting with them.

The sergeant warned me not to put holiday leave in. 'Just do it, Ash. And keep out of trouble.'

'Me, sarge? I don't know what you mean.' Like a truculent child, I knew exactly what he meant. Keep my eyes and ears focused on the job. No running off after someone, no nabbing shoplifters who just happened to run out of a shop and into my path, no being sidetracked . . .

'If you see anything, or get involved in anything, call for assistance for someone else to deal with it. You're not getting out of clamping,' he warned.

Clamps were huge things, all fangled metal and heavy, and I hated them. The objective was thirty a day but sometimes you did a few less, sometimes more. If you consistently did less, you'd get a bollocking. I tried to make sure I did what I had to do, but I didn't like it.

There was an art to fixing a clamp and some of the clampers had it down to nth seconds. They had a competition to see who did it the fastest. The officer posted with them had to write out the ticket as quickly as possible, slap it onto the car windscreen and then leg it. It pleased me to be posted with a fast clamper. I hated lingering. Once the clamp was on, the only way for it to come off was for the driver to pay the fine and then the de-clamping van would turn up and take it off. We couldn't. Or at least that's what they always told me.

If the driver of the car appeared before we left there was often a showdown. I had sympathy but, ultimately, they shouldn't have parked there. And they should have looked out for the clamping van. We took a lot of verbal abuse. Sometimes it was physical.

Like all cities, parking in London is very difficult and very expensive. If you find a space it's easy to overrun your meter by a few minutes. Some people took liberties and constantly parked where they shouldn't and they deserved to be clamped. Some folk, usually the yuppies, would deal with it as an occupational hazard. If they got clamped early in the day, they wouldn't phone up and pay the fine until much later. They'd treat it as a parking cost and put it on expenses.

If a vehicle was parked in such a way as to cause an obstruction, we would call the towing lorry who would turn up and cart the offending vehicle off somewhere deep in south London. I had less sympathy with them. It was difficult enough to drive in London, especially driving emergency vehicles through the packed streets. If you caused an obstruction, you were fair game to be towed. A few people reported their car as stolen only to discover it had been towed off. A sharp and harsh lesson.

Some clampers took great delight in finding expensive top-of-the-range cars to clamp, and those with exclusive private registrations. If they nabbed someone famous they'd lord about it for ever. The same with fancy cars. I hated being posted with that type of clamper. We'd spend most of the time in Mayfair and the posh streets of Westminster looking for the best and biggest cars. It drove me mad and those shifts were the longest.

Every clamp van had an hour for lunch. Police officers' breaks were constantly interrupted; you always had to be ready to drop-and-go in an instant and you frequently didn't get a break. It was different on the clamp van. They always had a full hour. You'd either get 12–1 or 1–2 for lunch, varying it to fit in with the second van. Except for Fridays.

Every Friday lunchtime the clamp van would travel to Lambeth, pull up outside a grotty little pub and park alongside the clamp vans of other local authorities, builders' vans and other assorted lunchtime drinkers. I suspect some CID from nearby police stations may have imbibed too, back in the day when lunchtime drinking was almost a convention.

I'd buy a takeaway coffee from the tiny café opposite the pub and sit in the clamp van with my sandwich, bag of crisps and an apple while my clamper would enjoy his hour with colleagues. I'd read the tabloid newspaper bought by the clamper that morning and I'd skip over the pages of bare-breasted ladies. I'd get ahead on the paperwork while he'd be in the pub watching the strippers.

I hated my time clamping and was so glad when I never, ever had to do it again.

Willy warmers

It's cold on night duty. Freezing on occasion. I suggest thermals. Or thick tights. But being cold was not the reason I was knitting at four in the morning when posted as station officer.

I was station officer because I was biding my time, waiting for my posting to Surveillance and trying to keep out of trouble. I'd already had a month on the dreaded clamp van and now it was my turn on the front desk. This included fielding the drunks, redirecting the lost, and taking reports from those wishing to make complaints of thefts or lost property. After midnight it usually fell quiet.

My case files were up to date and the correspondence in my tray had been dealt with, as much as it can ever be. I'd read the daily bulletins and made regular cups of tea for the custody office and CAD room, the hub of the station where all messages were received and allocated, hence Computer Aided Despatch. I'd checked the missing persons binder and the lost dogs, of which there were none; the kennels were empty. My thumbs had been twiddled until they were sore.

As night duty was a week long, it became boring. By Wednesday I decided to take in some knitting. If I followed the pattern, I found it was one of the few craft-like things I could do without winding myself into a knot. I was knitting baby clothes for a friend of mine who was pregnant. Little mittens, socks and baby cardigans are small, easy to do and quick to make, an ideal filler during the night once the city had settled down.

At 2.30 a.m. a call came out about a disturbance in the upstairs room of an exclusive restaurant in the St James area. It was a private party that had ended with a family at war – drunken, argumentative and causing a breach of the peace. Five men and one woman were arrested. The rest of the party turned up at the front desk, irate, drunk and demanding solicitors. They insisted their loved ones had to be released, now, this instant.

My attempts at calming them down failed. The sergeant in the CAD room heard the raucous carry-on and came to my assistance. Two of them ended up arrested for causing a disturbance and swearing at the sergeant and me. One of the remaining crowd tried to reason that his family had been falsely arrested. I listened, nodded and asked him to take a seat while I made tea and coffee for them while they waited for news. Feeling generous, I threw half a packet of digestives onto the tray too.

By 4 a.m., those in the cells were sleeping, as were some of the rabble loitering in the lobby.

One of the arresting officers, Joe Fenelli, stopped by the front office for a coffee and a chat. I was busy – knit one, purl one, knit one, knit two together – working on the sleeve of a baby cardi.

'That's them settled down,' he said. 'All over a bit of posh totty.'

I laughed.

'What you knitting, Ash? Willy warmers?' he asked, pulling a thread of wool.

'Hey, get off!' I tugged it back. 'Yeah, I got white, lemon and baby blue,' I joked, knit knitting away.

The following morning some of the prisoners went to court for breach of the peace and the others were kicked out, sheepish and hungover.

A couple of weeks later I was issued with a Regulation 9, a form 163, that the Complaints Department (now Professional Standards) issue to give notice that someone has made a complaint about you. Everyone on duty when the Hooray Henrys were arrested was served with a 163. The whole shift had been subject to complaints from the wealthy and influential family. The allegations comprised a variety of things including unlawful arrest, insubordination and abuse of force. Mine was for 'performance of duty' issues.

It was alleged that while on duty I was knitting willy warmers, neglecting my post when I should have been conscientious and diligent. What nonsense. I couldn't believe it. And to think I'd been kept inside the station to keep me out of trouble!

An independent panel was convened to interview every one of us.

'Officer, why were you knitting at five a.m. in the morning?' said the chap on the left.

'It was four o'clock, sir. And I took my knitting to work because it was very quiet and nothing much was happening.'

'During work time, officer? Surely there was some paperwork you could do? We're always hearing about how much paperwork there is these days.'

I confidently told him, 'All my paperwork was up to date, sir.'

He looked surprised.

The woman on the panel looked down her nose at me and said, 'What exactly were you knitting, miss?'

I hated being called 'Miss'.

'Baby clothes, ma'am. For a friend. One of my colleagues, PC Fenelli, joked I was knitting willy warmers but I wasn't, it was a baby cardigan.'

The older man on the panel woke up and said, 'Willy warmers? What are they?'

No one answered.

I filled the uncomfortable silence by adding, 'I was knitting the sleeve of a baby cardigan, sir. It can become tiring on night duty when you're posted to the front desk. Nothing much happens past two in the morning during the week but we still have to man the front office. I hadn't had a refreshment break and you can't really expect to be relieved for an hour by another officer when it's so quiet indoors and they are busy out on the streets. I sat and ate my sandwiches and did some knitting at my desk during what would have been my break.'

That must absolve me, surely?

I was wrong.

The lady of the bench glared at me. 'Could you not read law books? You don't know it all, officer. There are plenty of updates and changes in policy and law to become familiar with, I am sure.'

My quiet protestations of, 'But that would well and truly put me to sleep!' were ignored.

They had me.

I was given words of advice and told that in future I should read Blackstone's police manuals during the nights when I was bored.

And to think, I'd given that family our last packet of biscuits. That's gratitude. It put me off knitting, too. I never did finish those willy warmers.

Cut!

A few days after the willy warmers' incident I was back on day shift and still station officer. I made the tea and coffee, checked my handover files and offered to do some typing for one of the dyslexic blokes on shift who was bogged down with his paperwork. I liked to do a good turn and as a quick typist it earned me a few favours in the bag.

I hoisted the manual typewriter onto the counter and swept to one side the bundles of flyers and vouchers that littered the front desk. These comprised the usual advice leaflets for those who find themselves homeless, for domestic violence victims, plus some small street maps and handouts for new restaurants and fancy cafés that enticed customers with generous discounts in return for reviews. Theatres did the same to fill seats at preview shows. A pair of tickets for a West End show cost just a pound. It wasn't a gratuity because these offers were given to all offices, hotels and shops around the West End and were meant for all to enjoy the perks, police and public alike.

A flyer for Vidal Sassoon salon in Mayfair fluttered down to the floor. I picked it up. 'Models Wanted. Free haircuts.' It sounded perfect as I was thinking I could do with a new style for the new job. I phoned and booked my free cut for Thursday, 3.30 p.m., after the early shift finished.

Thursday was uneventful on the front desk and I arrived keen and eager at the hairdresser's. I signed the consent form, rather chuffed to be having my hair cut at a place I would never usually be able to afford. I skimmed the small print and sat down, unconcerned. It's only hair, right? It grows back.

My hair was shoulder-length with layers of rotten half curls, hanging limp at the ends. It was time to shed the remnants of a shaggy perm. I needed a new look. Being out of uniform meant no more pinning it up beneath a police hat and it could fly free.

Hairdressers from all over the world came to Vidal Sassoon to be trained and to learn new techniques. A male hairdresser from Chicago was assigned to me, under the guidance of Gideon, his tutor.

'Perfect!' said Gideon. 'And you've agreed the terms? That we can do whatever we like? And take pictures to use in advertising if we so wish?'

'Oh yes, I'm quite looking forward to it,' I smiled.

He didn't smile back. 'As long as you're prepared. There's no going back. And no suing us.'

'Absolutely,' I nodded, a tad too trusting.

The two men tugged and pulled my hair and entered a technical discussion that was beyond my ken. I started to feel a bit concerned as they discussed how my hair needed treatment to gain back lustre.

I glanced to my left and saw a beautiful girl in her early twenties with long blonde hair and symmetrical features. She could have been a model. Might have been a model. A real one. I felt a tingling creeping up the back of my neck when I saw her hairdresser take a razor to her head. She was being scalped! It was only then it dawned on me that I wasn't going to be given a conventional cut. Oh dear. Could I take my leave?

When I came back from an intense conditioning treatment, my

pretty neighbour was all-over bald. I could have cried for her. I couldn't understand why she was smiling. Maybe she wanted a total change. Maybe she had been given a modelling job, or was an actress that needed a bald head for the part? Maybe she had cancer and wanted it cut off before it fell out?

I felt uncomfortable as I glanced away and out of the window. I noticed two of my uniformed colleagues talking to a motorist who did not look happy. I shrank further down in my chair, hoping they wouldn't glance in and see me.

A rumpus erupted outside and the suspect ended up with his arms behind his back, handcuffed.

My hairdresser picked up his scissors and watched the commotion. 'I see cops are the same on both sides of the pond, honey,' he drawled.

'Mmm.'

'Too many innocent motorists getting popped when these guys should be out catching real criminals,' he said, chopping a wedge from my hair.

'Mmm!' I didn't like the way this conversation was going.

'At least your cops don't have guns, like ours.' Chop. Chop.

'No, that's a good thing,' I agreed, glad of something positive to say.

'You'd think they'd have better things to do than hassle people parking for too long. Not as if he's an armed robber, is it?' Chop. Snip. Hack.

I bit the inside of my lip. Who knew what they were arresting him for? He might have committed murder for all we knew.

'Who would do a job like that? Sick in the head if you ask me.'

I didn't ask him but maybe I was sick in the head – for agreeing to be a patsy for a hairdresser from a fancy salon.

'So honey, what is it you do?' he asked.

Wide-eyed and impotent, I looked back at him from the mirror in front of me. I tried not to notice my depleting locks.

'Oh, I work in an office. Just around the corner. Boring, nothing exciting,' I spurted out, coward-like and quivering.

'Let's see if we can liven up your life a little then, yeah? I think a streak of purple at the front with a long fringe hanging to the side. Short at the back.'

I tried to avoid looking out of the window. I didn't want anyone to recognise me and wave. I didn't fancy being a baldy or having any other revenge cut by someone who loathed the police.

I was relieved when I saw the van pull up and take the prisoner away. I relaxed a little, until I looked in the mirror. What the hell had I agreed to?

I left the salon with dark purple hair, which I had to admit was better than one streak, but I'd certainly stand out working under-cover with this colour. I doubted my boss would be happy. It was chopped short at the back and the hairline was cut fashionably raggy, according to Gideon. I had a long pointed fringe that hung down to the right but as I'd forever had a right-hand parting, never a left, it felt odd. I didn't suit my hair hanging down and for years I'd worn it behind my ears, not in front. If I were little instead of large, I'd have looked like an elf.

The salon photographer had taken a couple of pictures and I have no idea if any were ever used. I've never had the stomach to look in any hairdressing magazines.

The next day I took a trip to my regular salon and had it tidied up, which is what I should have done in the first instance.

Therein lie a couple more of life's lessons:

1) Sometimes it's necessary to lie and 2) there's no such thing as a free haircut.

House bugs and other nasty things

There is so much to learn when working undercover, aside from surveillance techniques. Of course I'm not going to reveal tactics and practical working methods, though I'll let you into some of the more interesting aspects of the job. But first, before any of that, there is a huge amount of law and protocol to understand and adhere to. If you don't know it, you can't work with it.

RIPA, The Regulation of Investigatory Powers Act, 2000, governs the use of covert (undercover) operations. Prior to RIPA, 2000, permission for such jobs fell under different regulations, but today these operations require the highest authority. Chief constables are vested with the power to authorise officers to use directed surveillance, to tap phones, intercept mail and email, to put bugs in houses, cameras in offices and so on. It has to be necessary and either in the interests of national security, for the prevention and detection of crime, or to prevent disorder or otherwise in the interests of public safety. There are other reasons but these are the main reasons police use such operations.

Chief constables delegate to high-ranking senior officers, normally the head of the crime department, a commander or chief superintendent, or whoever the relevant force policy dictates at the time. The sorts of offences investigated using covert surveillance are serious crime such as murder, paedophile rings, high-scale drug dealing, major fraud, armed robbery and national security. It can prove and disprove someone's guilt. It's expensive and time consuming, the operations long and arduous. And it doesn't always bring results. Before resorting to covert surveillance methods evidence should be gathered another way, if at all possible.

Barristers and judges are, as you would expect, hot on RIPA and the use of it. It has to be sound, justified and significant. It will be tested in the courtroom and evidence will be dismissed if it hasn't been gathered and recorded correctly. There is no room for error.

Specialist officers are assigned to plant the bugs, cameras and other devices. Justifying the expense is a major headache for the budget holders and, of course, it is a factor that influences decision-making. The easiest, and probably cheapest, method is a phone tap. A boring job but someone has to do it, listening in to phone calls.

House bugs helped us to secure a conviction for a couple that had systematically abused their baby. The father got a life sentence when the child died and the recorded conversations in the couple's kitchen were invaluable in proving his guilt.

Phone calls nabbed a national paedophile ring that planned to kidnap a nine-year-old girl.

Many a bad cop has been rooted out through intrusive and covert surveillance and in those cases the judge highly commended the use of covert ops.

The general public think the police can do more and know more than they actually do, so if you think they're watching you, they probably aren't. But it might be the DSS, or the NHS, or the Tax Office, or the Local Authority, or Customs, or one of many other organisations covered by RIPA . . .

Who's there?

When I joined the surveillance team I found that undercover work is 90 per cent boredom and 2 per cent action. But, oh, what action! The other bits of the job involved meetings, briefings and admin. We did a lot of sitting around in cars. We would sit up in buildings, on park benches, and traipse and trawl the streets. Occasionally we had to mingle, mix with suspects, and pretend to be someone we weren't. It was a bit like acting, but not at all like it's portrayed on the screen. It was also dangerous and addictive and far from a nine-to-five job, or foot patrol.

Surveillance units function locally, regionally and nationally, often overlapping, working together on joint operations that include phone tapping, house bugging, following people and accessing information on suspects, as per RIPA and other legislation. Our job was to gather information, intelligence and evidence, to find out what we could about suspects, the things they did and who they mixed with, and also to build up a profile of them. Sometimes we'd be given dossiers on criminals and we had to do the rest of the legwork, tracing and tracking them and monitoring their every move. We didn't often get in on the arrests, either. We would assist these bigger inquiries and investigations and pass the information back to source once the objectives were achieved. We also worked on our own cases. And although it could be monotonous, trailing someone who didn't do much for hours, you always had to keep sharp. A foot wrong and cover would be blown; you'd lose the whole thing, making it a costly and botched operation.

A lot of long hours are spent working closely with colleagues of the opposite sex. You're in situations where you have to depend on each other entirely and trust is essential. It's not unusual to form close friendships that, even if innocent, threaten personal relationships. The unpredictable lifestyle, having to drop everything to go off on a job, not knowing when you'll return, can be a strain. I was fortunate, I suppose, that during my years working undercover and in plain clothes, I didn't live with a partner.

One guy I was seeing became very jealous and suspicious. He wasn't a police officer and didn't understand why I couldn't refuse when I was called into work, or why I didn't want to say no. Neither did I wish to discuss my job with him. He accused me, wrongly, of having an affair with a married colleague. I became so sick of his accusations that one night, when I was paged at 10 p.m. to go into work, I left him in a bar and never saw him again.

It's well known that police officers deal with high levels of stress and alcoholism. I've known a few alcoholics in the job. One detective had a large bottle of water on his desk and it was only when the DI ordered him into rehab that I realised it was neat vodka. Another detective would leave me to work alone on night duty because he couldn't do without a drink. If there was a major incident I had instructions to call him, otherwise I was on my own. It was sort of accepted practice. He was a good detective with a vast knowledge and great way with people. He was a lovely man. Like many, he was a functioning alcoholic. I was upset to find out he committed suicide when he was forced to retire after thirty years' service.

Ronnie was someone I worked with undercover. He was married with three little boys. I went to see his wife when their youngest was born. They were a beautiful family. I didn't question Ronnie on how he knew where all the drug drops were going down, or why he was always disappearing off to see an informant. I didn't ask any questions when he came into work beaten up. He was rarely partnered with me, but one time when we were posted together I noticed he was acting strange. I thought he'd had a drink but couldn't smell alcohol. After an hour, he had a call from an informant and he went off for the rest of the shift. I was on my own for the remainder of duty.

A few months after this, Ronnie was arrested. He'd been under surveillance by Complaints. I don't know if he was criminally prosecuted, but he was sacked for malfeasance in office, a catch-all for officers doing wrong. Ronnie was addicted to heroin and had got himself into a right mess with the wrong people. Despite all my knowledge about addicts, I'd never guessed. Alcoholics and other addicts learn to hide their addictions well.

Another colleague, Ben, ended up as a resident in the mental institute where we often took patients. He was signed off work with stress and had become so paranoid that he was convinced he was under surveillance by some secret squad. He phoned us to report exploding pavements outside his house, insisting they were coming to get him. The sergeant sent Barry and myself to go and see him.

A paving stone had lifted from the pavement and sparks were shooting up from beneath it. We called the gas board and the local council. They came to fix a problem with some underground pipes but Ben remained convinced someone was after him. He was in such an agitated state we had to call his doctor who ended up sectioning him. It was very sad, especially when his wife left him.

Some officers went so deep undercover that they ended up

being arrested along with the suspect groups they were infiltrating, unable to blow their cover and often part of the overall strategy, because if they did end up nicked, it could only help keep their cover. Then there are those more recently in the media who formed relationships with the people they were supposed to be working against. I don't condone this, but I can understand how it might be easy in those circumstances to forget the boundaries after a long period so close to those people.

Someone I worked with went off on a long-term drugs operation in Manchester, or Leeds, or another big northern city. He was shot in both kneecaps when it went wrong. He had to take medical retirement but was lucky he wasn't murdered. Another undercover officer had a concrete slab dropped on his head. He suffered permanent brain damage and had a drastic change of personality. He also had to leave the service.

Police departments operate within geographical boundaries, unlike criminals, who don't. Surveillance takes you wherever the suspect goes. My work took me all over London and up and down the country. I loved it, all of it, but especially the undercover part. There's nothing to beat it. I did miss nicking burglars and general villains, reporting the neighbour disputes and stolen cars and rolling around with drunken street fighters on a weekend. The transition was difficult to begin with, having to switch off and ignore calls about that sort of stuff. From time to time we did stints in the CID office and it was good to touch base, to be reminded of how people lived their lives in the real world. You can't live in the deep and murky underworld too long. It's not healthy.

The following is a selection of some of my good and some of the not-so-good escapades undercover. I hope you enjoy them as much as I did.

In the crowd

When you work undercover you work in teams. It wasn't uncommon to make a three-pronged attack on an unsuspecting suspect, and sometimes it might be four or five or six of the team tackling a group. More often, though, it's just two of you.

My regular partner was Barry. We were a bit of an odd pairing. He was a good few inches shorter than me and ten years older. He was married with kids and I was single. Neither of us were favourites of the sergeant in our unit at the time because we didn't fit the mould of 'jobs for the boys'. He liked 'yes men' and we were not. He thought Barry was too old and he didn't like female officers. He thought we were a drain on the team because, in his words, female police officers were either bikes or dykes, too pretty or not pretty enough, and high maintenance. The sergeant was someone who liked the perks of the job and neither Barry nor I enhanced that. At least we knew it wasn't just us; he was quite irascible with many others, too. Still, you can't get on with everyone.

I think he thought it would be funny to put us two together, setting us up to fail. We might have looked a bit like the odd couple but we had the last laugh because Barry and I got on great. We had such rapport. He was gentle, funny, rarely moody, and when he was I would laugh at him and he'd do the same for me. I was quite serious and he lightened me up. There was never any sexual attraction and that helped us work well together. He was like the older brother I never had. I don't think I ever had a falling-out with Barry. Maybe we did, because everyone does, but if so, it must have been insignificant because I don't remember. We made a good team.

There were a dozen of us on our squad and the sergeant made thirteen. We worked hard and played hard. The hours were long and often stretched into the next day. We spent many hours in clapped-out cars, empty buildings, bustling cafés, and on the heaving streets. Ten hours would pass as we watched and waited and nothing would happen. Then we'd go from nothing at all to all-out action in seconds and we had to be prepared: no sleeping on the job, no skiving, no blinking, in case you missed something.

If we were lucky, we'd have one radio between two of us. And sometimes none at all, as you will discover. If there was a demo on, or some other big uniform operation, there wouldn't be any radios left so we had to rely on our wits. If we expected trouble, we'd have to try to secrete a truncheon somewhere. We didn't have body armour, or CS, or guns, but we had handcuffs and warrant cards and that had to do.

For bigger operations, we had earpieces and microphones, but it wasn't the norm, they were the exception. When all the criminals had mobile phones, we had pagers and our own crude way of keeping in touch. But it seemed to work. We had some good hits. We learned our craft and did the job, all the while mingling in with the crowds. And whereas you'd never get three uniform bobbies on the beat together, we often worked best in a trio, covering all angles.

As you'll see, Barry and I dealt with a lot of offences, and there are usually only three reasons for a crime. Money. Drugs (which includes alcohol). Sex. There are always exceptions, but I bet you find elements of one or all at the root of most offences. I don't generally believe in a motiveless crime, but then I love the psychology of people and I'm always looking for a reason why. And that's why I loved my job.

Fast forward

I like to think I'm open-minded. I try not to criticise people's lifestyles and I believe that to understand someone you have to walk in their shoes. A cliché perhaps, but working with the public brings you into many different lives and it's not for me to judge them.

The only way to learn is by example, by experience (yours or others') and knowledge. Knowledge is power. I hadn't realised how naive I was. The first preparation I had for working undercover was a major eye-opening experience.

It was a hot sweaty day, a boring day, and I sat in a stuffy room at Bow Street Police Station. There were half a dozen of us and it was the first time I met the guy who was to become my partner in crime – Barry.

The instructor broke us in gently. He made us watch a snuff movie.

Then he showed us various clips of sadism and masochism. One guy hung naked from a telegraph wire, large butcher hooks through his genitals and each of his nipples. Then came examples and photographs of auto-erotic asphyxiation – one man strangling another to near death, another man with a plastic bag tied on his head, a Chinese man hanging himself from a staircase and his partner cutting the rope at the salient time. Extremely risky play for the ultimate sexual satisfaction and sadly, in some cases, accidental death.

Women were not exempt. There was a woman choked by a penis and another woman branded on her clitoris while wearing a deep-sea diver's mask. Why?!

One man was bound like a prize piece of meat in the centre of the table, complete with an apple stuffed in his mouth. He was a major figure in business, apparently.

More peculiar predilections came after lunch, for those of us who could face food.

There was the fat man who liked to dress as a baby and be whipped with a cat o' nine tails, the woman who masturbated while a man tattooed her nipples, the group of men fastened together by a chain attached through their penis rings. One gave a tug and the others whimpered in distressed delight.

When I thought I'd seen it all, some of the worst was yet to come. Bestiality. Child porn. And a ritualistic child murder by a paedophile ring. Horror, revulsion, disgust, creating visions in my head.

It was a couple of weeks later that I went on my first sex shop raid. It was interesting, the first time. The feeling soon waned.

We seized drugs, counterfeit goods and a quantity of under-the-counter videos in brown envelopes. The number of smart-suited men that came to the door while we were inside was astounding. It was obviously big business, the sex trade.

I guess you could call it equality when the sergeant gave me the bag of videos we'd seized and said, 'There you are, Ash. The next three nights taken care of.' He was serious. And it was most definitely business. I had more than fifty cassettes to check for hardcore and/or illegal porn. If the shopkeeper was selling stuff with kids, snuff movies or animal porn, we could prosecute him and close the shop down. We already had him on the drugs, and Trading Standards were investigating the fake bedroom toys.

The way to check the videos for evidence is by watching them on fast forward and silent. Some things were easy to spot – those obviously underage, the blatant sex acts with animals – but the borderline age of consent and the pseudo snuff movies were difficult.

A lot of the films were grainy, difficult to see on normal speed never mind fast, so it was a case of stop, rewind and watch again, this time closer. Some of the films had been recorded, re-recorded and copied again, so the quality was very poor. A lot came from Eastern Europe and beyond. There were a number of Japanese films of a dubious nature.

Every cassette had to be checked. Sometimes the label would give the title of an all-action movie or recent release, but dodgy recordings would be put in the middle and the video passed off as a regular film. Just when you thought you were watching the latest Bruce Willis, twenty minutes in and a porn flick would pop up. They would last a few minutes and then it would go back to the regular film. It might happen once, twice or many times throughout the tape and it was a common tactic.

Some films were old, some homemade, some professionally shot. Some were a few minutes long while others seemed to last for ever. Many were the same movie in different cases and various states of quality.

It's boring and tedious to watch porn films on fast forward in an attic room of a police station on night duty on your own. Not that I wanted company. By the end of the third night I'd watched all fifty videos. There was a handful I considered borderline child porn. It was difficult to say if the youths were under or over eighteen. I wasn't happy calling it so I let my male colleagues decide. The rest of the batch, although distasteful, appeared to be within the law, though some things made my eyes water, even on fast forward.

It was a grim job, but someone has to do it. And it was good experience for when I went to work in Child Protection.

Working the streets

Until you get good at undercover work you're a bit rubbish. You make mistakes, trip up and stand out.

It was very much a dress-down job, unless of course you had to dress up. You wore whatever you had to fit in with the job in hand. I usually wore jeans, T-shirt, maybe a jumper, flat shoes for running and something to put a radio in, such as a jacket or a bag – somewhere suitable to hide it. Soho is great for covert places to loiter – lots of café bars, shops, and street corners to hang around on without attracting attention.

I was walking up Rupert Street with Barry, my partner in crime. It was one of our first times together and we were both new to it. We had information about a guy allegedly dealing drugs on the corner of Greek Street. It was a light evening, the night young. The Raymond Revue Bar was beating music onto the worn warm streets as we headed towards our destination. It wasn't that busy but it wouldn't be long before the area filled up, buzzing with vibes and drink and heady tourists looking for excitement.

I became aware of a short stout guy bumbling towards us. Barry and I parted to let him pass between us. I moved to my right and the guy moved with me. I was about to move the other way, like strangers dancing on the pavement do, being polite to let each other pass, when the guy shoved his big fat shovel-hand between my legs and gripped tight. His fingers squeezed and I jumped back. I shouted out and grabbed him by his open shirt. Barry jumped on his back and between us we grappled him to the ground. Barry put him in a headlock.

The sickly smell of alcohol oozed through the man's skin and curdled my stomach. His breath was sour, his face ruddy and his eyes wobbled in his head. He was drunk, your honour.

'You're nicked ya dirty pervert!' shouted Barry.

I could feel the man's hands as if they were still touching me. I called for a police van, still in shock at the cheek of the guy.

Alberto José Menezes went to Bow Street magistrates' court charged with indecent assault. He represented himself and pleaded guilty. The magistrate asked if he wanted to say anything in mitigation.

My jaw dropped when he said, 'I thought she was a prostitute. How was I to know she was a cop?'

He was fined £100 and ordered to pay £40 compensation to me.

'It would have been cheaper to go to a prostitute. And I'd have got a lot more for my bloody money,' he grumbled.

Six weeks later I received a cheque from the court. Mr Menezes paid his fine straight away, cash. I felt I needed to do something significant with the money.

I bought a new pair of work jeans.

Bit of a handful

Huge crowds gathered outside Planet Hollywood for the grand opening. Like bees to pollen, it was an ideal playground for thieves as they hovered over tourists: rich pickings. Six of us, Gary and Pete, Matt and Max, me and Barry, joined the throng on the look-out for familiar faces and suspicious individuals while the crowd waited for a glimpse of Arnie, Bruce and Sylvester, the Hollywood stars.

Security men stood in the doorway pushing people back but still they spilled onto the roadway. We stood at the back of the crowd, watching, waiting.

We'd been there half an hour and it was hot, sweaty and boring. I glanced to my left and saw a six-foot-tall man on his own, looking at the crowd, focusing just on females. I saw him creep behind a young woman. He didn't try to steal from the bag slung over her shoulder but he pressed his body against her back and jerked his groin into her. She took a few steps forward but didn't turn. I watched him stand behind another female who didn't seem to be aware of the man behind her. His hands were punched into his jeans pockets, knuckles straining at the denim.

Yes, I knew what he was up to. He was a pervert.

I nudged Barry and told him to watch the guy with the blond floppy hair and haversack on his back as he moved into the crowd.

We moved either side of him and watched as he took his hands out of his pockets to hover over the buttocks of a small female with long dark hair. I couldn't see if he touched her as his body was so close to her and the person in front of me not only obstructed my view but stank of garlic. I'd just inhaled a waft.

Less than a minute later our suspect moved near to Barry, his hand hovering by the trouser-clad bottom of another small dark-haired female.

She moved to her left; maybe she'd felt something that prompted her to shift her position. She glanced behind her and he stood there, looking straight ahead at the doorway, apparently oblivious to her. Both sets of body language suggested he'd touched her, but in a jostling crowd it happens that people accidentally brush against one another. It would be easy to excuse it and I was sure that would be his explanation if we challenged him.

He stood there for a few minutes and I watched his eyes wander across the crowd. He settled on a brunette standing on her own and he made his way towards her.

I knew from experience that it could take hours before the celebrities made an appearance for a few short minutes. And it could take ages before we had enough to arrest our man. Barry tipped the others off about our suspect but Matt and Max had spotted a face in the crowd, a handbagger (bag thief) who they were concentrating on, and they went off to follow him up Regent Street.

Barry, Gary, Pete and I positioned ourselves at four points around Mr Touchy-Feely. He might have been a genuine odd-bod but I doubted it. I was confident he was there for a specific purpose and it wasn't to see celebrities.

He stood behind the woman he'd been watching. I saw his right hand move to her buttocks. I wasn't close enough to see if he touched her or if he was merely floating his hand. She flicked her head and her hair swung into his face. She turned, smiled at him, and I saw her mouth, 'Sorry.' She moved away, probably thinking she was in his way.

We watched him approach a number of different women over the course of half an hour and I had no doubt about his intentions. We decided we needed a different course of action. We had to speak to the women.

It was disastrous. Two couldn't speak English. Two hadn't been aware of him at all and another had seen him but hadn't felt anything. One refused to have anything to do with us and another ran off crying.

As we had no victims and no independent witnesses, we couldn't prove a thing. There was only one thing for it.

I positioned myself near our man. I moved myself towards him until I stood directly in front of him. I was there for a couple of minutes when my right arm jolted forward. I turned and saw the couple next to me vying for a better position, pushing their way to the front. I waited. I flicked my hair. I looked at my watch. I waited. And I waited. I didn't turn around. I didn't want him to acknowledge me as that would put him off and he'd move on.

It was nearly two o'clock. The crowd was dense. I was thirsty, hot and a bit bothered. People are very smelly in close proximity. I waited some more.

Then it happened. I felt it. A touch. On my bottom. Between the cheeks and between my legs. Although I'd pre-empted it, I was still shocked. I turned and shouted, 'Oi!' I grabbed hold of the man and he stared, two golden eyes round and large, surprised at being challenged.

Barry and Pete stood either side of him. They pulled him out of the crowd, two burly undercover coppers with a pervert in a headlock. I held up my warrant card and people parted the way, allowing us to pass through. Good timing. The celebs arrived as we took our man out, and the screams and hollers increased as we left Coventry Street. We were ignored in the commotion.

We took our prisoner into the station to great protest. He cried. He could barely speak, snot, tears and saliva running down his face as he gave his details to the custody sergeant.

He gave his name as Jason Mountford, aged thirty-three and living in a flat in Islington. When it came to searching him, Mountford asked if I could do it but I had to say no as male prisoners have to be searched by male police officers.

When Barry and Gary came out of the detention cell having completed the search, I realised why he'd asked for me. He was embarrassed. Underneath his jeans and T-shirt he had been wearing five pairs of female knickers and a bra.

When Barry and I interviewed him it was apparent Jason Mountford had a number of issues. He'd been cautioned ten years earlier for flashing in a swimming pool but had kept out of police trouble since. He said that for as long as he could remember he'd struggled with his identity but he always knew he liked women. He was an emotional wreck. He admitted to touching all the women we asked him about and then some more.

We charged him with indecent assault and he remained in custody until his court appearance the following morning. I felt a bit bad and not just because I was a victim. He seemed in need of treatment rather than imprisonment, which I suspected he might get. He was a good-looking man with problems that wouldn't be solved in prison because I suspected he'd have a very hard time of it and very little support or therapy.

Once we'd finished the paperwork and processing of our prisoner, Barry, Gary, Pete and I went for a debrief drink. It was busy and loud. Tina Turner blasted from the speakers. I stood at the bar getting the round in as I thought of Jason Mountford.

I wondered if he was still crying. Something, someone, pressed close behind me. I felt a touch, a light caress on my bottom, just like the one I'd felt earlier that day. I didn't move. I deliberately didn't look. I stepped forward. It was my turn to order the drinks.

Sewer rat

You might think the streets were paved with paedophiles and perverts but that's not really true. I did begin to wonder, though, when one Sunday night six months after dealing with Jason Mountford, I was indecently assaulted again.

I was late leaving work because I was dealing with a prisoner. I sank into Piccadilly Circus tube station around eleven thirty and apart from two station guards, it was deserted – the buskers gone, the tourists in bed or in hotel bars, and the tube tunnel mice were getting ready to come out to play. The air was muggy with the tangy steel of tube trains, old dust and the stale odour of people.

I stepped onto the escalator, bone weary after a hard week. My rucksack was slung over my shoulder and I felt it jostle. I turned and there was a guy stood close behind me, invading my personal space. I stepped down a couple of steps and leant against the rubber handrail to steady myself. My bag shifted again, fell off my shoulder, bashed against my leg. Panic gripped me when I felt a hand on my bottom and one creep around to my chest. I almost toppled from the step as I turned and pulled away from the guy. He had a wild look in his eyes like a madman.

'Help! Help! Help!' I screamed as he lunged over me. A rush of adrenalin pounded behind my eyes making my head hurt. I didn't have a radio to call for assistance but it wouldn't have worked deep down in the tube station anyway. I glanced up and noticed we were the only two people on the escalator in either direction.

I grabbed the man's arm.

He reached out his other hand towards me and squeezed my breast. I struggled with him, all arms and bags and moving staircase. I tried shouting but the words stuck in the back of my throat. I couldn't scream, just like it happens in those nightmares when the words don't come but you try so hard.

He touched my face and I pawed him away but tried to keep hold of him at the same time. I wanted to run but didn't want him to get away. As I couldn't scream I started to spit but I had no saliva. 'Pah, pah, pah.' It was a bizarre thing to do but all I could manage.

We reached the bottom of the escalator and I stumbled over the sudden stop. We both teetered but I held on to him. He leant towards me and I smelt an overpowering sweet smell, stronger than aftershave but not poppers, which is sharp. It was a mixture of sherbet, sickly fruit and over-fragranced flowers.

We fell to the ground, him on top of me. My knee buckled and a sick feeling flipped in my stomach. I retched, in pain, in fear and fright. What if nobody came? What if they'd closed the station and we were the last people here? What if he dragged me through the tunnel? Horrible thoughts filled my head.

Then I heard the thundering of a thousand boots. I thought it was in my head as I lay on the dirty floor, stunned. A dozen hands like bird's claws flew down and lifted the man from me. Someone helped me up.

I admit, for a moment I was frightened. I wasn't such a tough guy, or a tough bird, after all.

A traveller at the top of the up escalator had seen the man touch me the first time and heard the kerfuffle. He'd alerted the guards who called the police and it had been captured on the station's coarse CCTV.

Simon Farquhar Brown didn't go to court. He was suffering a mental disorder and was sectioned. He should be pitied. I'm not ashamed to admit that he frightened me. You can't reason with or fight a madman.

In true police fashion, I was ribbed. It was part of the banter, part of the healing process, brave camaraderie. But some things stick. I don't like being the only person left in the building. I dislike taking the last tube or bus home unless I'm with other people.

It could have been much worse. I'm glad it wasn't. We can all be victims of crime, even those of us who work to prevent it.

Suspects with benefits

There were far fewer female officers than males and I don't want to get into the realms of sexism because things have changed. It was just the way it was back then and there were some tasks that only women could do. I don't mean making the tea, though for a long time it appeared thus.

Some jobs were gender-specific, like searching prisoners. This meant that whenever a male officer brought in a female prisoner, the whole station was searched for a WPC. I've even known the female chief inspector be asked if she'd mind searching a prostitute. And why not? Though I can imagine what some of the male chief inspectors would say if asked to search a rent boy. And the answer would almost certainly end with '— off'.

I happened to be in the station writing up an arrest for a pair of handbag thieves Barry and I had nicked that afternoon. The phone in the canteen rang and rang and because I could never leave a phone ringing, I answered it.

'Oh, Ash! Good. Can you come and search a prisoner?' asked PC Brown, the gaoler.

Mumble, grumble and of course, I had to go. I could say I was busy but once the custody sergeant knew I'd been found, if I said no he'd be ordering me down. And I didn't mind, not really. We had to help each other out and yes, it was a bind, it interrupted my work, but it's what we had to do. And it was nice to have a favour in the back pocket should I need one later.

The arresting officer, PC Jenson, told me he'd arrested Julia Macintosh for possession of cannabis and causing a disturbance. She'd been arguing with a punter in the street and threatened to smash his face in if he didn't give her another twenty quid. I knew Julia and felt sorry for her. She was forever being beaten up, ripped off or caught shoplifting. Another sad tale of someone coming to London in search of their fortune. She'd come to escape her father and brother who had both sexually abused her for as long as she could remember. I'd tried to encourage her to report the historical abuse but she never would.

'Okay, Julia,' I said, pulling on a pair of rubber gloves. 'Anything I'll find?'

'Nah, only that spliff he took off me,' she said, clacking chewing gum.

'You'll have to spit that out,' I said, holding up a rubbish bin.

She looked as if she was going to protest but I shook my head and pointed to the bin. I was surprised the custody sergeant, Bob Chamberlain, hadn't made her get rid of it but he was busy and every cell was full.

I took Julia into the fingerprinting room and asked her to remove her outer clothing. I patted her down, searched her pockets and her shoes, and then she took her jeans off.

There had been a fire in a cell recently due to a female prisoner secreting a lighter in her underwear, so we had to be particularly vigilant when it came to searching. It was a job I always hated. Intimate searches for major drug offences were only carried out under specific authorisation and then only by a police doctor called for the purposes of an intrusive drug search. This wasn't necessary for Julia. A spliff didn't merit that sort of search. She had her back to me and I asked her to bend over. As she did, I saw a bulge in her pants.

I asked her to turn around and when she did, her pubic area was flat, covered by her white pants, but something poked down into the gusset.

'Okay, Julia. What have you got down there?' I asked.

'Same as you love. Only less bollocks.'

'What is it? You either give it up or we stay until the doctor comes and he'll get it.'

She crossed her legs and said, 'I've got nowt.'

Someone hammered on the door. 'You finished? I need to fingerprint and photograph my prisoner.'

'Tell the sergeant to call the doctor. I need an intimate search doing,' I called back, looking straight at Julia.

'Eh?' said the officer on the other side of the door.

'Just ask him to call the doctor. Please,' I shouted.

Sergeant Chamberlain burst through the door. 'What's all this? She doesn't need an intimate search.'

'She's got something in her knickers, sarge, and she won't give it up. I don't fancy rummaging around in there so it'll have to be the doctor,' I said.

'For crying out loud, Julia. What've you got? I haven't time for this.' Bob Chamberlain stood, hands on his hips, his face worn and tired.

Julia stood in her pants and T-shirt, arms across her chest, staring us out.

Bob reached up to the shelf, grabbed the box of rubber gloves and pulled out a fresh pair. He snapped them on.

'Hey! Hey! What you doing?' said Julia, pulling her T-shirt down to cover her pants.

'The doctor's busy. Needs must. If you don't give it up . . . well, you don't leave me an option,' he said.

'Okay! Okay! Get out! I'll give it to her,' she shouted, pointing at me.

'Two minutes. I'll be back.' Bob Chamberlain left the room.

'Perv,' whispered Julia.

In one swift movement she pulled down her pants and grabbed the bundle hanging down from her vagina. She threw it across to me with a snarl. 'There, satisfied now?'

I caught the roll. As I opened it out I saw it was a DSS benefit book. The name on the stub was Michelle Delaney.

I cautioned Julia and asked her what she was doing with someone else's benefit book.

'Minding it,' she said.

The benefit book was stolen but we couldn't prove Julia had nicked it. She was cautioned for possession of cannabis for the spliff, and charged with handling stolen goods.

Julia was kept in custody and went off to court the next morning. As was required, I was there too, 10 a.m. sharp. I was glad when Julia pleaded guilty because I didn't fancy explaining it all to a bemused jury. She was given bail pending a pre-sentence report. As she walked past me out of the court, a look passed between us, an acknowledgement. We'd never be best friends but we had the cohesion common between regular petty crims and cops. I wished there was something more I could do for her, to help her get out of the lifestyle, but I knew she'd have to reach out and help herself first.

Summary justice

We worked hard on the squad and our bosses expected good results. The hours were punishing but the job worthwhile.

At Christmas the streets were rife with handbaggers and pickpockets so every December we were tasked with a three-week spell of twelve-hour days, no time off.

The thieves often worked in pairs, threes, sometimes fours and hung about in cafés in places such as Hamleys, Simpsons, Fortnum & Mason and the Royal Academy on Piccadilly; places where the pickings would be worth it. The MO is simple. People leave handbags hanging from the backs of chairs or lying on the floor by their feet. It's easy to slip a bag away and it's surprising how many people don't notice.

We posed as customers, spending up to an hour or more in one place, waiting to recognise a face, an action, or spot body language between the small groups who would operate in these locations. We knew what we were looking for if not always who. To a trained eye, they become easy to spot and it was all part of our education. That and drinking lots of coffee while watching and waiting.

One afternoon we arrested a three-handed team for stealing a bag from a lady in a shoe shop in Oxford Street. She'd put it on the floor while trying on a pair of shoes. One of the team sat beside her and looped her foot around the bag handles. Another member took over and dragged it along the floor. The third one bent down, picked it up and off they went.

The suspects denied it, as they do. The case was listed for Great Marlborough Street magistrates' court in March the following year.

Their trainee barrister, Ms Fredrica Agnita, was pleased with herself when she wangled the case to be dropped on a technicality. I was fuming. We knew they were at it, had caught them red-handed, but our word wasn't good enough when up against a technicality. Barry and I left court to their grinning faces and the trainee barrister's smug smile.

Half an hour later, as I tried to explain to our unimpressed sergeant what had happened, control room asked us to go back to the court. They said there was a job they thought we should deal with.

Barry and I moaned all the way there, stomping through the streets in our best court suits. Probably some sort of disturbance. Surely it was a job for uniform? We were met by Ms Agnita.

'You?' she said, frowning when she saw us.

I had to try very hard not to laugh as she told us she'd been pick-pocketed by her clients.

'What evidence do you have that it was them?' I asked.

She blushed. It hadn't been caught on CCTV because the court didn't have any back then. There was no direct evidence because she hadn't seen them do it.

'One of them knocked into me on the way out. It must have been them.'

I couldn't help myself. 'But you've just told the court they weren't thieves.'

I took her report of theft of her purse from her bag, which

included all her bankcards and the £100 she'd taken from the bank that lunchtime.

'We'll arrest your clients but I dare say they'll deny it. After all, the court was busy this afternoon so technically there's any number of suspects. Especially as you didn't see who took it.'

She pursed her lips, seething.

I told her we'd be in touch.

Summary justice had never been so sweet.

Unmistaken identity

Barry and I had been to Crown Court and were pleased that a pair of thieves who had stolen the handbags from two ladies who lunched at the Royal Academy café had both been given a year's prison sentence. It was the thirtieth conviction for Ricardo Mendez who had been out of jail for just six months when we'd arrested him. His female co-worker was about to enjoy her first night in Holloway ladies' prison.

We had a couple of hours left until the end of our shift and were feeling buoyant and eager to get back out there, to maybe nab some more handbaggers, van-draggers or other criminals.

We changed from our court suits into street wear. As we were about to leave the station, the sergeant called us over, waving a printed CAD message at us. 'If you're going out, there's just been a smash and grab at a jewellers in Bond Street. Suspect is male, white, little, in his twenties, wearing a red baseball hat over ginger hair. He has one arm and a hearing aid. Shouldn't be too difficult to spot.'

'It's a wind-up, sarge, surely?' I said, laughing.

'Nope. That's the description the witness gave control room,' he said.

We set off on foot for the vicinity of Bond Street. Police patrols would be out looking for him but we knew the back streets and had the advantage of not being in uniform, so he wouldn't dodge us if he saw us coming.

Five minutes later a youth wearing a red baseball cap sauntered towards us in the midst of pedestrian traffic heading home. He was singing something very out of tune, one sleeve bunched into his bomber jacket pocket, and a thick gold link chain swinging from side to side around his neck. Tufts of bright ginger hair poked out from beneath his red cap. He was a little over five foot, looked about seventeen, and had virulent red spots smattering his cheeks. I saw a hearing aid over his left ear. As he walked towards us, I saw the sleeve tucked into his pocket was empty. He didn't have a right arm.

When we stopped him, he looked surprised. We arrested him on suspicion of burglary and took a wild guess that the heavy gold chain worthy of the wealthiest rapper and the three diamond rings he wore on the fingers of the hand he did have were the booty.

We walked him back to the police station and he bopped along beside us, quite happy to chat. He gave his name as Timothy Moore and his address was one of the young persons' hostels near Holborn.

He said in his mumbled and diffident way, 'How did you know it was me?'

I looked at him. 'Seriously? You fit the description perfectly. There aren't too many young men with red caps, ginger hair, a hearing aid and one arm walking these streets.'

'Maybe there is,' he muttered. 'People don't often notice me.'

Aww. I could have cried! Poor boy. I wanted to give him a hug and I couldn't help but feel a little bit sorry for him. It transpired he'd been in various foster care homes all his life. He had lived all over London, so hadn't had much in the way of continuity of health care and had dropped off many of the systems as they changed to computerised records. He not only felt invisible, but to society, despite his obvious look, he *was* invisible. He was just the sort of kid who needed good old-fashioned mother's love, not a young offenders institution where he *was* destined to end up. The cost of the theft was over ten thousand pounds. Ten pence, ten pounds or ten thousand, it didn't really matter to Tim, I'm sure it was all attention seeking.

There wasn't a lot I could do for him apart from call social services, who were the ones who'd arranged 'independent living' for him the minute he'd turned sixteen. Tim wasn't really bad. He wasn't really mad. It seems wrong to call him unfortunate, but I guess that's what he was. I hope it's different for him now.

Down the drain

Barry was on leave and I was working with another colleague, Matt. We worked well together and he made me laugh. We'd been keeping observations, or obs, on a couple of guys because we had information they were involved in dealing drugs. It was almost one o'clock in the morning and the suspects weren't doing much. I was tired. Another hour and we were going to call it a night.

The guys had coffee with some other men in a café in Old Compton Street. They then went to a gay club in Soho. Of course, I'd stand out if we followed them into the club and it would somewhat defeat the object of being undercover, so Matt and I sat in a pub opposite drinking lemonade, keeping an eye on the door for when they left.

One of our two suspects soon left the club and we set off after him. That's how they worked, a double-handed team, with their anti-surveillance techniques. One would leave and entice anyone watching to follow him. A short time later, the other one would leave, pockets full of tabs and pills and other drugs. What our clever suspects didn't know was that Matt had contacted our colleagues, Gary and Max, who were also on duty. They'd agreed to take up the obs inside the club whilst we watched outside, ready to follow the first man. They would be able to lift the second as soon as he left, probably about ten minutes after his pal.

They weren't clever enough to know that.

We followed our man to a bus stop in Regent Street. We had no intention of getting on public transport with him, so we made our approach. Matt told him who we were and I explained the grounds and object of the search.

He gave his name as Danny Lee.

'Yeah, yeah, I know the drill. I've got a tiny bit of blow. Personal use. Nothing else,' he said.

Matt searched Danny and found a small matchbox in his front left-hand trouser pocket. He opened it and inside the box was a lump of cannabis resin, enough for one or two reefers. Matt passed the box to me and somehow, between him handing it over and me taking it off him, the box turned. The resin tumbled out. Plop. Straight into a drain. Oops!

I looked at Matt. He looked at me. Bang went our evidence.

'Okay,' said Matt. He turned to Danny Lee. 'You didn't want to be nicked, did you? Consider this a warning. Next time, you'll be coming in.'

The night bus pulled up and Danny hopped on. As it drove off he gave us a grin and a little wave.

I waved back, our solace knowing his pal would soon be ours.

Doors

One hazard of the West End was that it was either very quiet or steaming busy. When it was that busy, prisoners had to be thrown in together because there weren't enough cells for one each. This particular night we had three or more prisoners to each cell.

The bottom cell on the left wing contained prisoners Steele, Graham and Anon. They'd all been drinking and had been arrested at different times during the night for minor street offences:

Mr Steele had been nicked for loitering for the purposes of supposed prostitution.

Mr Graham had been arrested for assault and possession of a couple of cannabis reefers.

Anon was a drunk and disorderly who refused to give his details.

It was only when the gaoler, PC Brown, a rather dour Scot, commenced the 4 a.m. cell check that he discovered the dirty deeds going on inside.

He lifted the hatch in the middle of the cell door and was faced with the back of a black donkey-jacket. He prodded the body wearing it, ordering the prisoner to move.

'Shift your arse,' came the technical term.

'Oh, that hurt!' came the retort.

'Move. Now!' barked the gaoler.

'Make me,' the voice shouted back.

Six foot and hefty, PC Brown was not to be messed with. He banged on the metal door, rattling the hinges, and hollered. 'If you don't move, we're coming in!'

Laughter and other assorted grunts were heard.

'Ahhh!'

'Ugg, ugg, ugg. Ooooh!'

Various insalubrious sounds echoed through the cellblock.

'Sarge, bring the troops!' PC Brown yelled, jangling the large metal keys on the ring hanging from his belt as he searched for the right one to unlock the cell door.

Within minutes, five officers disturbed in the middle of their refreshment break tumbled down the stairs from the closed canteen. They stood at the open cell door, mouths agape.

Mr Steele, with his blond, curly hair and a beard that looked like it was full of blackbird feathers, was bent forward accommodating Mr Graham, a thin, weedy middle-aged Mediterranean-looking man. Mr Anon was standing by the conjoined bodies; he'd obviously been pleasuring himself but was now inspecting his non-existent fingernails and shifting his broad shoulders beneath his too big jacket.

The three detainees said nothing, as if by magic struck dumb.

'Fetch a bucket of water,' barked the custody sergeant as the troops hesitated to pull the two men apart.

Night-duty CID were called. We scrutinised the law books.

A police cell wasn't a public place.

All prisoners were adults, all well over the age of consent.

None of them were making any allegations or complaints about the others.

They were all complicit.

We searched and searched, looking for every loophole we could think of, but even in spite of there having been police witnesses to the act, there was nothing at all we could do about this previously unknown-to-each-other ménage à trois.

All three were given stern words of advice, with butts firmly kicked out of the station once the morning shift had dealt with them for their arrested offences.

Three to a cell was never allowed again. Not in our police station.

Dead or alive

Barry and I had a warrant to execute in Sydenham. I wasn't familiar with the area and it was long before sat navs, but we did have a battered *A–Z* street atlas of London.

We found the address we were looking for, a large dilapidated Victorian-style hostel that had once been two properties but was now converted into one, housing many bedsits. It had five floors and a basement. The entrance had rows and rows of silver intercom buttons and we had no idea which one to press as they weren't numbered. Barry pushed the double front door and it swung open.

The lobby was dark and dull with a whiff of something bad in the air. A high desk like a lectern stood to the right. A sweeping staircase with a colourless carpet was in front of us. A couple of closed doors bore numbers daubed in permanent ink. The door immediately to the left was a common room. It housed a couple of scruffy settees, some tattered books, and a tiny portable television with a coat hanger aerial. The room stank of cigarettes and urine. I could imagine a vagrant wandering in, lying down, peeing himself and falling asleep.

'How are we going to find number thirty-six?' I grumbled to Barry.

'Dunno. I can't imagine there are thirty-six bedsits in this place,' he said.

We went upstairs. Eight. Thirteen. Sixteen. No reasoning to the numbers.

Each floor had a bathroom and separate toilet. All were soiled and smelly.

'I'm dreading what lies behind the doors of these bedsits,' I said.

'Yup. Typical inmate accommodation,' said Barry, trying a door handle.

Bail hostels, probation hostels, ex-cons, no fixed abode, including those vulnerable and in need of care in the community usually lived in places like this and it never looked much like caring to me.

On the next floor we found an open door. I peeked into the small room, no more than eight feet by ten. A single bed lay under the half-open window. The sheets were brown, completely brown, but weren't supposed to be that colour. They'd once been white. Or perhaps cream. You could see the shades of dirt, changing from fawn to dark brown. Even though the window was open, the room smelt foul. Rancid like the worst curdled butter and sour like the worst milk. And faeces. The room was littered with papers and rubbish and scraps of clothing.

Barry poked his head in behind me. 'There's a man in the bed.'

'I don't think so. It's just a huddle of filthy sheets,' I said.

'No, really. There's a bloke there.'

We walked across to the bed. Barry was right. There was a man. A little shrivelled-up old man, tiny, naked, skin and bone, and completely brown, for a white man. He wasn't moving.

'I think he's dead,' I said.

Barry put his hand on the man's chest. 'Yeah.'

'We'd better go get someone.' I tried not to gag as I left the room.

We ran, down the stairs, upstairs, throughout the whole building, but we didn't find anyone. We'd stumbled into a nightmare. I searched the lectern desk while Barry went outside to see if he could see a sign on the door or the gate that would give us a clue, or at least a phone number, for whatever agency ran the hostel.

Barry came back into the lobby, a strange look upon his face. 'Ash. We've got the wrong address.'

'What! What do you mean? We can't have the wrong address,' I said, mooching among unopened envelopes and junk mail. I didn't want to entertain the idea. He must be mistaken.

'It's the wrong address. Not the one with the warrant. We should be three doors down.'

Shit. Now what? We'd just illegally gone into a property we had no right to enter, but not only that, we'd found a dead body. How the hell were we going to explain this to our cantankerous sergeant?

We stared at each other, trying to think what to do next.

Finally, I said, 'Well, we can't leave him. We'll have to call the local nick. If anyone knew we'd been here . . . that we'd found him and left . . . besides, it'd haunt me for ever. We'll just have to think about the consequences later and hope nobody asks too many questions. And it *was* a genuine error.'

Barry agreed. 'It's not as if we've broken in, is it?'

Neither of us was convinced.

'Better find out who he is,' I said. 'Or was. How awful, to die like that, in that state.'

We walked back up the stairs, slow and heavy-footed, cursing our bad luck. We entered the room, trying not to breathe too deeply. We walked to the bed. We both looked at the wizened old man.

'How long do you think he's been here?' I whispered.

'Dunno. He looks like he's been freeze-dried.'

He did. A perfect description. I nodded. 'Yeah, like a locust.'

'Suppose we'd better call it in,' said Barry.

'Yeah,' I said, knowing neither of us wanted to.

I don't know why I bent closer to look at the body but I did. I put my face near his.

The body jumped.

I jumped.

I screamed.

Barry screamed.

The body screamed.

We all screamed.

'Wha' yo' doin' in my hoose! Gerrout! Gerrout!' the body shrieked from a black and toothless mouth.

We didn't need telling twice. We ran. Oh, how we ran. Better and faster than Scooby-Doo and Shaggy ever had. We ran down the stairs and out of the door and into the car. Barry started the engine, stalling it the first time. We shot out of the road and drove into the mid-morning traffic like we were being followed by a half-dead, naked, freeze-dried locust.

As the shock wore off we started to giggle until we both collapsed in laughter.

Barry had to stop and pull over. When we'd calmed down we both still felt quite bad about it. Poor man. Maybe he wouldn't thank us for our help but I said I'd contact social services and see if they knew about him, if there was anything they could do. Back in the office, when the sergeant asked how we got on, Barry said, 'Oh, it was a waste of time. No one home, all locked up, and no way to get into the flat. We'll try again, take the local beat officer with us next time.' Barry changed the subject. 'So what's this job Max is doing this afternoon?'

We spent a whole week worrying about the old man and worrying whether anyone would complain about intruders in a block of hostel flats in Sydenham. Nobody did to our knowledge. I contacted social services, out of earshot of the sergeant, but the hostel had that many itinerant occupants there was no way of knowing who he was or what help he might need. I left my contact details anyway.

The warrant went back in the drawer for another day.

The day I met . . .

Barry's sister was a dancer who worked in the West End. She often performed in theatres on our patch. One night after a good hit at Crown Court where a street-robbery gang had been sent down for twenty-two years between them, we went out to celebrate the positive result. Barry said his sister was going to a party that night and suggested we join her. Of course, the Crime Squad lads were eager to mingle with delightful dancers. It wasn't the first time they'd blagged their way into after-parties. We were usually made welcome and it was great fun.

This time there was only Barry and I left standing as the others had fallen by the wayside. We'd had a bit to drink, nay, a lot to drink, when we arrived at the club. Barry opened the door for me and we entered the heaving party. Then he was gone, no longer by my side, and I didn't know where he'd gone. I didn't realise there was a curved wooden staircase leading down to the basement bar area. I stepped forward, stumbled, and fell all the way down the stairs. I landed at the feet of a rather dishy young man who helped me up but didn't look impressed.

I smoothed down my clothes and ran clumsy fingers through my hair that was more bed-head than coiffured. I tried to smile at my hero but he'd turned away to talk to a guy at the bar. I was aware of glances, of staring eyes, tut-tutting and whispering. It made me nervous. There was no sign of Barry. I was a definite intruder. I searched the small crowd but he'd disappeared. I did the only thing I could do. I left.

The next day Barry asked where I'd gone when he nipped to the loo. He'd bought me a drink and waited for half an hour but I didn't show. I told him about my accident and he laughed. He said he knew the guy and that he was a friend of his sister. He was playing in *Phantom of the Opera* and was going places, apparently.

That was the day I totally embarrassed myself and fell for John Barrowman.

Street people

The streets of London are paved with chewing gum, muddy puddles and secrets. Forget the gold and promises of flashing lights because the reality is you'd be lucky to find a penny and the lights are usually emergency-service blue. The West End is full of pale grey buildings and strutting pigeons, and beauty is a by-product in the form of nostalgia and history.

Working undercover in the same area regularly means you become a familiar face to the street people. It doesn't take too long to be known and for the price of a pack of cigarettes or a cup of coffee you can find out most things. There was a sort of mutual respect and an unofficial rich source of information.

One female vagrant, Iona Donald, was a little ruddy-faced Scottish woman who looked like a drooping fuchsia; sort of pretty but far past her best. She was a rampant nymphomaniac who could take her pick of men like her as she was one of few women living on the streets and probably the only one who was up for satisfying their needs.

She laughed when we caught her at it with a fellow vagrant in St Mary's churchyard. She'd usually barter her wares for a can of Tennent's but told us she'd always fancied this one, Marcus, the son of an aristocrat. Marcus had a drug habit that had brought him to the street and when we spoke to him he gave us the name of a supplier who doled out cannabis and ecstasy to the school kids on tourist trips. It was a trade-off. We told them to keep out of sight in future, as we were sure they wouldn't want to be arrested for outraging public decency. They took themselves off to an alleyway behind the Raymond Revue Bar.

Dunkin' Donuts was a popular haunt for the street people, with the enticing smells of cinnamon that you could taste when you walked by and the sticky lemon icing that looked far too yellow and gooey, and the too strong coffee that burned if you spilled it before it was cool. It was outside Dunkin' Donuts that I met Michael DiMarco.

Michael was a good-looking guy in his late twenties, a bit taller than me, and very slim. He always smelled of soap. I knew he made use of various hotel facilities to wash and keep himself clean, which many of them did until they were caught and chucked out. His worldly possessions were rolled up inside the sleeping bag he kept tucked under his arm. I'd often see him outside the doughnut shop when I was on a 10 a.m. shift. It was his chosen corner. They all had them – open shop doorways where heaters would belt down comfort and warmth, places where unsuspecting tourists could be hijacked for a pound or two.

I saw Michael watching us when Barry and I arrested a pickpocket.

The next morning Michael whistled to me as I climbed up from Piccadilly tube station. I smiled and walked on by.

'Hey, copper. I've got your number,' he shouted. 'Me and you could do business if you're interested?'

I waved him away and continued down Regent Street.

Three nights later, Barry and I were hanging about Piccadilly Circus, looking for a thief who'd walked out of Simpsons department store wearing a suit worth over a grand.

Michael came over and said, 'I've got some information if you're interested?'

'What sort of info?' I asked, keeping one eye on the crowds.

'There's a guy who picks up young lads on the meat rack. The young ones, you know? I don't think it's right.'

Shaftesbury Avenue was where the artists sat touting the tourists and where young men touted their bodies. It was known in the trade as the 'meat rack'.

'What's in it for you?' I asked him.

Barry walked away, his interest taken by two guys who may or may not have been thieves. Or tourists.

'Nothing. I just don't like it. These kids on the streets being picked up by men like him. It's one thing living rough but them selling their underage arses for next to nowt isn't right. This guy, he's a big fish and well known.'

'Who is it?'

'Not prepared to say . . . not yet.'

'What are you after?'

'Meet me in the morning, buy me a coffee, we'll talk.' He reached out a hand and rested it on my shoulder. It felt intimate, strange, nice but not. I shrugged him off.

'I'm on another late tomorrow. Make it Thursday. I start at ten but I'll come in a little earlier.'

He smiled. 'Thursday is days away. I don't think I can wait that long.'

'You'll have to,' I laughed. 'I have to have some days off.'

He was easy to talk to, pleasant, articulate. I saw pain and hurt in his deep blue eyes and there was a secret. But they all had them. In the eyes. Always in the eyes.

Barry came back as Michael walked off. 'What you doing flirting with a tramp?'

'Behave. I'm not flirting,' I protested. 'And he's hardly a tramp.'

147

'He is. And he likes you. I can tell.'

'Give over, Barry. He only wants to pass on some information.'

'Yeah. To you, not me,' he teased.

Four days later I arrived at Dunkin' Donuts at twenty past nine. There was no sign of Michael.

I loitered for a couple of minutes. I thought of the paperwork on my desk waiting for my attention. I could make good progress with an early start. I walked off down Glasshouse Street.

Behind me I heard, 'Juliet Bravo! Juliet Bravo!'

I turned to see Michael. I couldn't help but return his smile. It was infectious.

I took him to a café just off Brewer Street. We sat at a table at the back.

He gave me the registration number of a private-plated BMW that he said belonged to the someone famous he'd mentioned the other night. Michael told me his name. A kids' hero. I agreed it could be *News of the World* material if the media found out. Michael didn't want anything in return except a cup of coffee and to be left alone on the street when he asked for a spare bit of change, guv'nor.

I asked him why he hadn't tipped off the newspaper because that's what most folk in his situation would do.

'You think they'd believe me? A homeless person? Someone with my history? Nah. I've seen you, watched you for months, know how you operate. You seem okay. I'd rather you nicked him. If the papers got it, he'd deny it. You lot can catch him at it. I hate them, the perverts. Especially ones like him. Think they can get away with it, buy their way out. He needs doing properly, arrested and banged away an' all that. Proper like.' He played with the plastic spoon in the sugar bowl, white sparkly grains scattering across the checked vinyl tablecloth. His eyes were not sparkling. They were dull. Dark and dull with his own secrets, which I suspected included a past of being abused.

There was a specific squad who dealt with juveniles, runaways and rent boys. I passed the information onto them. They were dubious when I gave them the name of the suspect but said they'd check it out.

I took Michael for coffee the next day to tell him it was now in the system.

Whenever I was on a 10 a.m. shift, I took Michael to the café and we'd talk. He told me about his alcoholic and abusive stepfather. About his mother who worked all the hours she could until one night her husband beat her so hard she fell down and died. Her death certificate said heart failure. Michael said his stepfather had broken her. He didn't know his real father so he was put into care, abused by the system and those who were supposed to look after him. He fell into crime and charmed his way into fraud school and a jail sentence. His girlfriend didn't want to know when he came out of prison, so he had nowhere to stay and he ended up on the streets, no job, no home and little money.

He give me snippets of information, such as where a posse of handbag thieves left their stash of empty bags and nicked purses; told me of someone who dealt drugs to youngsters, of a guy who gave hooky notes to the bureau de change office, and the cashier who was in it with him. In return I bought him breakfast and gave him the odd few quid. I passed on all of his information and he proved to be correct.

It was good to talk to someone with a different perspective on things. He was intelligent and funny and sad. It was a most unusual friendship. He suggested we took a trip to the National Gallery one day when I wasn't at work.

'After all, it's free,' he laughed. 'And warm.'

'Maybe,' I said. Nice idea but I wasn't sure it was very ethical.

I took two weeks off in March and spent long mornings in

bed and long nights catching up with friends. I didn't buy a newspaper and didn't watch much television.

I returned to work the first Monday in April. Michael wasn't at Dunkin' Donuts. We hadn't arranged anything but I expected to bump into him during the course of the day so I trotted off to work.

I was first in the office, Barry was next. He took his coat off and after the 'Hi, how are you, how was your break?' he said he had something to tell me. I wasn't prepared for it.

Michael was dead.

Apparently, allegedly, he'd nicked something from a shop and had been chased by a security guard. He'd run onto the street and in front of a car and was killed outright. A head injury.

No. No! How? Michael never stole. He begged a little but he never stole. He couldn't be dead. It can't have been him.

'It was, Ash. It is. His sister identified the body,' Barry said.

I struggled not to cry. He was just a snitch, a grass, nobody to me. Not really. But he was. He was my friend.

'He didn't have a sister,' I said.

'He does. She's arranging the funeral.'

I refused to believe it.

'How well did you know him?' Barry asked, caring but not understanding.

'Well enough.' I knew he didn't get it.

'I've got her number if you want it. Ring her?'

I shook my head. My eyes stung but I wouldn't cry. My chest hurt, tight. 'No. After all, he was nothing to me, was he?'

Barry didn't answer.

I was given a paperwork day and asked to do some research on some suspects that had cropped up recently. I was kept busy, out of the way and occupied.

I didn't know Michael, not really. But he was somebody,

whatever his past. I don't believe he was a bad person. Not many people are, not really.

The man in the private-plated BMW never came to public notice. He was spoken to after an 'event' but never prosecuted and never exposed.

I watch and wait with interest. I know, one day, he will come.

Poisoning pigeons

There's many things they do to probationers. Cruel? Perhaps. Character building? Intentionally, yes. Piss-taking? Most definitely. Of course it's done in a number of professions but the police force is particularly harsh. I'm sure it's not as bad as it used to be on the grounds of discrimination and health and safety and all that, but a lot of fun has been stopped as has, rightly so, cruelty to animals. These things usually took place on night duty, away from prying public eyes and when the streets were quieter.

During one of my stints between working in CID, I was posted as night-duty detective. It was a break from the daily grind and I missed working nights. During the quieter hours if there were no serious crimes to deal with, it was also an ideal opportunity to catch up on paperwork and do some research into those jobs that demanded a little extra attention.

There was a probationer who I shall call Carys. She was a lovely lassie from the banks of the River Dee. She was great fun, a good laugh and a hard worker. I miss her smile and her company on a good night out. On any night out!

When she'd settled on the relief, the term for the shift, there usually being four, A, B, C and D, and was considered familiar enough with everything, it was time for her initiation. She knew it was coming, only she didn't know what it would be.

I went on parade with the relief. At the start of each shift as you go on duty, the sergeant briefs everyone together on any important events or information, any current wanted people believed in the area, tells you your beat and what time refs you take. This is 'parade' and technically where the sergeant can ask to see all of your equipment and inspect your uniform and if you don't have it, well, you should. Punishments vary from making the tea to serious trouble for persistent offenders. As night-duty CID I decided to parade-on with the relief as it was my old shift.

They were given their postings and the intelligence reports were read out. The sergeant, Nick Dorman, posted himself with Carys, the first phase of the plot.

He called us all to attention and said, 'Listen in guys, there's been a spate of pigeon poisoning and they need to be culled. There's too many for pest control so they've asked that if we see any birds suffering from apparent poisoning, we capture them. As they're vermin, it's a case of extermination. Quick, methodical, clean.'

I stood in the background as the diligent officers wrote it up in their notebooks.

Sergeant Dorman said, 'If you see any ailing pigeons inform me straight away. I'll keep a tally and if we aren't tied up, me and Carys will come and do the deed.'

I couldn't look him in the face. Neither could anyone else.

PC Johnson piped up, 'I remember the last time, sarge. Spent all night duty chasing around trying to catch the pigeon.'

Cue Muttley impressions.

The sergeant turned to me. 'Didn't they catch someone for it last time, Ash?'

Crikey! Don't involve me! 'No, still out there somewhere, sarge.

We thought it was some suspicious seed but couldn't prove it. Maybe a rogue pigeon-feed seller in Trafalgar Square knocking it to the tourists. Could be he's come back. I'll take a pootle around when it's quiet.' I thought I did well to get out of that one unscripted.

It was a fairly busy shift and I had prisoners in the cells to interview and a file to write up. I forgot all about pigeons until I heard a radio message just after 4 a.m.

PC Johnson radioed up Sergeant Dorman. 'I've found a sus pigeon, sarge, at the back of the Regent Palace Hotel.'

Sergeant Dorman, his voice full of joy, replied, 'Excellent! Keep an eye on it. We're on the way.'

Poor Carys was turfed out from her break to deal with the poorly pigeon. No one wanted to miss this and, surprise surprise, there were many officers loitering around Dunkin' Donuts and the RPH, as it was known.

A poor pigeon was hopping along the pavement, close to the building. It had a leg missing and a broken wing hanging down one side. Half of its beak had broken off. I suspected it had done battle with a cyclist or a taxi. It didn't look well at all as it shuffled over to a vacant air vent chucking out heat. It was huddling and shivering and looked in agony. Poor thing.

Sergeant Dorman and Carys approached, both armed with large Metropolitan Police plastic property bags. Carys also clutched the force-issue evidence labels and a ripper seal, which was a vicious-looking plastic-toothed thing.

'Got your truncheon, Carys?' Sergeant Dorman asked her.

'Yes, sarge,' she said, pulling it from her skirt pocket. The shiny stick of wood looked pristine and ready for action as she held it up, raised in her right hand.

She still didn't realise what she was supposed to do.

'Go on then,' Sergeant Dorman said.

Carys stood back as a patrol car pulled up. Two officers climbed out. Another two on foot patrol who should have been on refs turned up. Then one of the vans appeared.

Carys stood there. She looked at the sergeant. Looked at the pigeon. She stepped forward a fairy footstep. The pigeon looked up at her with big sad eyes.

'Go on then,' Nick said again.

Carys held the plastic bag up and moved towards the pigeon. It fluttered further against the wall.

The sergeant shouted, 'Use your bloody stick!'

'I can't!' she squealed, though she did manage to put the evidence bag over the pigeon's head.

A mass of fluttering, flapping and fussing followed. Those watching were rolling about laughing. One officer leant against the wall, holding his midriff. Another had a fit of the giggles. It wasn't pretty. It wasn't nice. But the pigeon was in the bag. The sergeant grabbed the bag and bundled it into the back of the van, climbed in himself and slammed the doors. There was a lot of banging going on from inside. He shouted out a few times and the van rocked a bit. Then he climbed out without the pigeon. He spoke to the driver who sped off up Glasshouse Street.

Poor Carys was sent back to the station to write up a report about the incident, about how the pigeon looked, the evidence of poisoning, her actions, and how it all ended. She was told to fax it across to the Stray Pigeon Department of Westminster council.

Of course, she couldn't find the fax number so her report was left for the early-turn shift to send.

Carys got it back the following night, attached to a report from the relief inspector informing her it had all been an elaborate wind-up. To put her mind at rest, he said the pigeon had been driven to Hyde Park and released, away from the hustle and bustle of truncheon-wielding coppers.

Written at the bottom of the report was – '*No pigeons were hurt in the making of this wind-up.*'

'Ere!

When you work undercover the idea is that people don't know who you are or what you are up to, so when you chase someone and you're in need of a bit of assistance, the general public think you're fighting, or have been mugged, and they usually stand and stare, or walk on by and leave you to it. A bit like when you're in full police uniform.

Barry, Gary and I were the team and we were keeping obs in the Bond Street area where fancy buildings housed designer shops and expensive jewellers. There had been a spate of high-value thefts in the previous few weeks and shopkeepers were becoming anxious.

You can tell a genuine toff, an aristocrat looking for expensive trinkets, and you can spot the rich customers by their shoes – smart and highly polished – but it was becoming increasingly difficult to spot the common thieves as the shabby chic mingled with the rough and ready. They didn't always dress for the part.

We struck lucky when a guy we'd seen enter a tiny jewellery boutique ran out a few minutes later being chased by a panic-stricken retailer.

Gary ran over to the shop and confirmed a theft. 'He's stolen a Rolex! Stop him!'

Barry and I gave chase but the crowds hindered us. I lost sight of the suspect for a minute but caught him again when I saw his bleach-blond head bob into an alcove.

'Over here, Barry!' I yelled, pointing to an office doorway.

Unfortunately, the suspect turned, looked at me and started running again. He was slight, only five foot six or so, and thin, so it was difficult to keep him in focus.

I watched as he ran onto the kerbside to dodge a group of Japanese tourists.

I heard Barry shouting behind me, 'Police! Stop that man!'

I was close, in reaching distance. I gained a few metres, reached out, touched the suspect's arm. He turned, looked at me and pulled away, stepping onto the road. It was then I noticed his right ear was missing.

I shouted out, 'Stop! Stop! Police!' and pulled my warrant card from my jeans pocket in the hope someone might help.

I became aware of a car, a white saloon edging down the road alongside me. The engine revved.

The suspect ran up onto the pavement and danced down the kerbside again.

The car sped up and mounted the pavement, driving straight into our suspect, knocking him over.

The guy fell, sprawled out across the pavement. I knew by the sickening angle of his leg that it was broken.

Barry ran from behind me and took hold of the suspect in case he decided to get up but he was going nowhere, unable to leg it.

The driver of the car got out. 'Are you okay? I saw you chasing him. Did he steal your bag? Did he hurt you?' he asked in a gush of gabbled words.

'No, I'm all right. I'm a police officer. We were chasing him. We think he stole something.'

'Oh! Right.' He paled. 'I'm not in trouble am I? For running him down? I thought you needed some help. You're not going to arrest me?'

'No, don't worry. Bit unorthodox, running someone over, but you stopped him. Thank you. We'll need a statement so don't go anywhere.'

Gary joined us with the shopkeeper, who thankfully identified our suspect as the thief.

Barry called for uniform assistance, as we now had a traffic incident, and he called for an ambulance, too.

The Japanese tourists stood around us, flashing their cameras.

Our suspect, Jonathan Keane, lay on the floor, swearing, threatening to sue everyone – us, the driver who ran him over, and the tourists taking photographs.

Keane was arrested and cautioned for theft of a £24,000 Rolex watch. Barry pointed out a Rolex on the prisoner's left wrist and a silver digital watch on his right.

'It's my watch,' Keane replied. 'They both are. I like to keep good time.'

Keane went to hospital under police guard and two hours later he was in the station protesting his innocence. After we'd interviewed and charged him, I almost felt sorry for him when he said, 'I should give up. Last time I was nicked I was only caught because some other bloody do-gooder ran me over. That's how I lost me ear.'

He went to court and pleaded guilty to the theft of the Rolex. Because we'd retrieved the watch and Keane had said sorry, and also because he'd ended up with a broken leg, he didn't go to prison. The judge gave him a community service order and a final warning that if he was found thieving again, no matter what the cost of the item, he would be going to jail.

The driver of the car was awarded £100 out of public funds and his local newspaper called him a hero.

I never came across Keane again and I hope for his sake it was because he gave up crime. He might not have survived a third good citizen.

Expensive jackpot

One sunny Saturday afternoon Jas, the other female on the squad, and I, were on were on general undercover patrol hanging around Piccadilly Circus. We were occasionally partnered together and between us we knew a lot of criminals local to the West End.

We'd given up on two suspects we'd been eyeing for the last hour in Leicester Square. They'd gone in and out of shops, picked things up, put them down, jostled a few customers, and generally acted like prats. Maybe they weren't pickpockets or handbag thieves and were just idiots.

We were considering where to go for our refs, which we usually took while out and about on the ground and keeping a close eye on the crowd. Jas wanted a burger but I was all burger-ed out. I fancied a sandwich and as it was a nice day wanted to sit by Eros and see who wandered by. I won the rock, paper, scissors battle and had just taken a bite from my pastrami on rye when I heard shouting. I looked up to see a young couple in their late teens arguing.

'No. No!' the girl shouted. She was little, with black curly hair, quite pretty, and very upset.

The lad with her looked angry, his cheeks red and his strawberry blond hair shaggy around his face. He was thickset and six feet tall, wearing a growl, all of which made him look thuggish. He was pulling at her sleeve.

She had tears in her eyes. 'No. It's mine. You're not getting it. It's my birthday money.'

'I told you, the machine's about to drop. I'll share the winnings with you. Give it to me.'

She shook her head and turned to walk away from him.

He yanked her backwards by her hair, a big clump of black curls held tight in his fist.

I looked at Jas. We were in civvies and didn't really want to blow our cover but this guy was nasty.

'Bitch!' He spat in his girlfriend's face.

It was enough. I shot up off the steps of Eros and shouted at him. 'Leave her alone!'

'Fuck off. What's it got to do with you?' he snarled.

I whipped out my warrant card. 'I'm a police officer. Get your hands off her.'

He let go of his girlfriend, flung his hands up, and in one smooth motion smacked his head down into my face.

I heard the crunch before I felt the sickening snap. My front tooth broke in half. Blood poured from my mouth and my nose, pooling beneath my tongue, which was now far too big for my mouth because I'd bitten it on impact and it had immediately swollen. I couldn't help swallowing my broken-off piece of tooth.

In Piccadilly Circus itself, probably because it's a major tourist attraction, there are plenty of people who might come to the assistance of those in need. They didn't know I was a police officer but lots of people tried to help. I was grateful for the crowd who wouldn't let the guy leave when he attempted to run off and Jas couldn't hold on to him. Friendly MOPs (members of the public) are a great help at such times.

Jas handcuffed the guy and we marched him to the nearest

police station, escorted by a furious crowd of MOPs, all willing to give statements about what they had seen Stuart Wilton do to me and his girlfriend. Of course, there were twenty statements of varying accounts of violence and aggression and I was more than pleased when Wilton pleaded guilty to ABH at magistrates' court.

He cried when standing in the dock. He was very, very sorry. His girlfriend had left him and he was now undergoing anger management and counselling because he realised he had a problem.

He was given community service and fined £500, which he had to pay to me as compensation. His father, I heard from my inspector in a confidential aside, was a police sergeant in a station somewhere deep in south London. He paid the fine immediately, no doubt horrified by the actions of his son. Another consequence of addiction, in this case gambling and fruit machines, is that it can turn unwitting people into criminals. I'm sure Stuart Wilton regrets his actions today.

Keeping up appearances

There was a girl I regularly dealt with in the West End. I'll call her Rachel. She was pretty with brown curly hair and a nice smile. She spoke very well and came from a different sort of background to most who find themselves on the streets.

Rachel was fourteen and one of the youngest of the girls that hung around Soho. She came to our notice because she was regularly reported missing by her parents who had a large apartment in Mayfair and a huge house on the south coast somewhere. Rachel had a place at an esteemed fee-paying school in Westminster and a life many would envy, but whatever was going on at home was prompting her to run away time and again.

I found her in doorways curled up in a sleeping bag with cardboard for a mattress.

I found her hanging around the meat rack, the archways in Shaftesbury Avenue, trying to convince the young boys not to sell their bodies or their souls.

And I found her walking around the empty city streets crying tears of rage and anger and sadness.

Rachel rarely spoke of her parents or of why she ran away. Maybe she kept quiet because of her father's position of influence.

Maybe it was to protect her mother. Perhaps it was to protect herself.

One day I found Rachel within an hour of her being reported missing. I knew where she usually hung out and I struck lucky. She had a black eye, which was fresh. She refused to talk about it.

'I'm going to have to report it to social services, Rachel. Especially as this is the fifth time in as many months that you've run away. Something's going on. What is it?'

She wouldn't meet my eye. 'Nothing.'

'You can tell me. I can help you.'

'No. No, you can't. Nobody can help. You think this is the first time the social services have been called? They won't do anything and it will make it worse.'

'I promise we can help.'

'You can't. I spoke to a teacher once and my dad got her the sack. He has power and influence and people listen to him. You can't do anything so I'll just keep running away until they can't find me. One day, nobody will find me.'

I made a report to social services but I don't know what, if anything, came of it. Rachel still kept running.

I found her with cannabis. I took it off her and gave her a talking to. I told her she was wasting her life taking drugs.

I found her drunk. I arrested her. Her father came to the station with his chauffeur. He was far from happy because he'd been pulled out of his club and a dinner with an important person who he alluded to as being the Prime Minister.

When I hadn't seen Rachel for a few weeks, I hoped she was okay. We hadn't had any missing reports and maybe it signified things had settled down. No news being good news and that sort of theory. It wasn't long after that I was called to attend the nick one night.

Rachel had gone with her mother, Dorothy, to the police station and they refused to speak to anybody but me. I was agreeable to come and see them but they had to wait for over an hour before I could get there.

They waited. Dorothy was a timid mouse of a woman. She wore expensive make-up and sported a bulging black eye, which was closed up but weeping tears and blood. Her nose looked broken. She sat in one of our plastic police chairs, whimpering like a little dog.

It took me more than half an hour to find out why they wanted to talk to me. I made hot sugary tea because they seemed to need it and Dorothy finally relented. She started to talk, unravelling the life I'd suspected they lived.

'He books my hair appointments, my facials, my manicures. He needs to know where I am, you see. It's his job, he has to know who I'm with at all times. He needs to know how I spend his money and I have to give him every receipt. Two pence adrift is enough . . . enough to make him angry. He thinks I've been secreting money away. Every penny has to be accounted for.' She paused and took a sip of tea. 'He makes his chauffeur take me everywhere. I can't go anywhere without Fred. He watches me and I know he reports back. Poor man, he has to do it.' She sipped some more. 'And I know my husband has other women. I smell them on him.'

Rachel took her mother's hand.

Dorothy whispered, 'He beats me.' She winced in pain as she held her ribs. 'He laughs at me when he hurts me. He splits my skin and he breaks my bones. And he's cruel. So very cruel.'

Rachel looked at me. 'I hate him!' she spat.

Dorothy eyed her daughter, disapprovingly or with dismay, I wasn't sure. She shook her head, little light curls bobbing but remaining in place. A waft of expensive hair spray drifted my way and I had no doubt she was a regular at some top Mayfair salon.

Dorothy continued, 'If I leave him, he will kill me. He's already threatened to ruin me. I have . . . I am . . . nothing without him. It would wreck his career if I were to leave.' She blew her nose into a paper tissue and winced.

It must have been excruciating. I saw the pain flicker across her face, a dark shadow of hurt. I watched mother and daughter, not sure which one was the strongest or the weakest.

Dorothy sat upright. 'The displays of affection in front of our friends, it's just an act. Everything about him is an act. He thinks everyone loves him, the comedian, the funny guy; the one with his hand in his pocket buying drink after drink. But they don't really. Do they? Like him?'

A rhetorical question I didn't feel the need to answer. I'd met him.

'Keeping up appearances, that's all,' she sighed.

'Do you have anywhere you can go?' I asked.

'You don't understand!' shouted Rachel.

'It's okay, Rachel. I'm telling her.' Dorothy took her daughter's hand and squeezed it.

She faced me, her closed eye weeping, her broken nose running, something I wasn't sure about in her eyes.

'Rachel said I could trust you? That we should only speak to you.'

'Yes, you can trust me. I can help. If you want me to. But I might have to discuss some of it with others.'

'I understand.' She paused. 'He came home tonight. Drunk. He'd beaten me before he went out, I can't remember why. The shirt he wanted wasn't there, or something. When he came home, he tried to embrace me, to slobber his bulldog kisses over my face. I pushed him away, a reflex. He revolts me when he's been drinking and I couldn't bear it. He teetered, just a little, swayed back and fro just once. But he's ever so cumbersome. He reached out to the banister and he stepped back and he lost his footing. There's such a drop to the floor from the top of our staircase. You've been into our apartment, haven't you?'

Rachel cried out, 'It was me. Me! It wasn't Mum! I pushed him. I pushed him down the stairs. It was me! Me!'

Dorothy shook her head. 'No. It was me. I didn't know he'd fall like that. He was drunk.'

'Mum, you don't have to do this. It was my fault.'

'Please, take no heed of her. She's trying to protect me. Like she always does.'

'Where is he now?' I asked.

Dorothy stared with her one open eye. 'On the floor. He's dead.'

I contacted all those I needed to and called a solicitor for Dorothy. She made a statement on tape in the presence of her legal representative. We didn't interview Rachel. She was too distraught and kept trying to tell us she had killed her father. Nobody believed her. We all knew she was protecting her mother and wanted to take the blame herself, for so many reasons.

The chauffeur made a statement saying his boss was drunk. Fred said he saw him miss his footing on the marble staircase and described how he tumbled down the stairs, arms over legs over barrel-belly.

He confirmed Dorothy had pushed him away from her but that it wasn't at the top of the stairs; it was on the landing. He said his boss had turned to march off downstairs and it was then that he fell, missing his footing. Fred said he knew his boss to be violent towards his wife and his daughter and had witnessed many incidents. He told us that what happened that night was an accident.

The coroner recorded a verdict of misadventure. The newspapers didn't speculate. The case was closed.

Rachel never ran away from home again. I'm sure today she's somewhere being a successful woman. I really hope so. She deserves it.

Marshmallow surprise

I was single, twenty-six, and couldn't believe my luck when Tig Turnbull, the detective with film-star looks and a great customer manner, stopped by my desk and flirted with me.

We'd worked together for nearly a year, me as the trainee and he, the older, experienced cop of thirty.

I blushed as he twinkled his blue eyes at me. His square chin and dimpled left cheek added to his boyish charm and I swooned whenever he passed by. Who wouldn't want some attention from the best-looking bloke in the office?

Once five o'clock struck, pending prisoners in the cells, the CID staff adjourned to the local hostelry. It became a habit, Tuesday to Thursday inclusive.

At the end of the evening, after many beverages had been consumed, the usual suspects were left – the singletons and the long married. Late one evening the only people left were Tig, myself and boring Phil, he with the halitosis problem. Tig had been on top form all night and it was with ease that he bent to kiss me on top of my head, all sloppy and drunken, as he swung out of his chair and wove past me to go to the loo. I sat in anticipation of his return, hearing nothing of the slurred conversation from our gooseberry colleague.

When I found myself on the last tube north instead of east, it seemed the natural and right thing to do.

Tig shared the top-floor flat of a Victorian semi with a colleague from another station. It was the typical male boudoir – assorted furniture, no matching cups, and piles of wet laundry slung over radiators and backs of chairs. Tig handed me a slug of whisky in a fancy cut glass while he disappeared off to his room, no doubt to tidy up and throw dirty pants, socks and T-shirts under the bed along with his stash of mild porn.

Tig and I enjoyed our time together, three nights a week for nearly a month. We kept our little fling hush-hush. Thankfully, although Tig was a ladies' man he was also known for his discretion. It all added to his appeal and charm. I didn't want the rest of the guys to think I was easy or the girls to think of me as another Tig Turnbull victim.

One of the guys in the CID office was getting married and arranged a stag night in the centre of town. No girlies allowed – none from work, anyway. Strippers were obligatory for a policeman's last ball whether the stag wanted them or not. Never one to miss a lads' night out, Tig was going.

A friend of mine suggested an evening out in town, so I arranged to stay in the section house accommodation that was available to us when we had long shifts and early starts. For a small fee we could stay there on the occasional night for social-domestic-pleasure reasons. The six pounds were worth it!

Tig had said he might drop in if it wasn't too late and I hoped he would. Blokes shouldn't stay over but we were all adults and blind eyes didn't see what went on unless there was trouble.

About one in the morning, after a great night out with Della, my old pal from training school, I fell into bed. There was no sign of Tig and I was a tad disappointed but I soon fell into a woozy sleep.

At three o'clock I was jolted awake by hammering on my door. Disorientated, I reached for a towel to protect my decency. I opened the door to Tig, wobbling against the doorjamb and smiling his lop-sided grin. He was very, very drunk, complete with whisky breath, stale smoke and cheap stripper perfume. But that cheeky boy smile won and I didn't have it in me to refuse him a bed.

Discreet as ever, we still hadn't told anyone what we were up to and arrived for work separately the next morning. I was first in the office and expected the guys to be late and hungover. Sure enough, they filtered in, bleary eyed, unshaven, with ruffled bed hair and stinking of sour beer.

As the post-mortem of the night before took place, I made cups of sugary hangover tea. Tig was the focal point of conversation. Tig, the strippers and something about marshmallows. The tops of my ears reddened as I stirred the teapot and listened intently while pretending not to as Phil regaled the story to an avid audience. Apparently, Tig had climbed up onto the stage and danced with the delightful ladies who had parted company with their clothing, piece by small piece. Okay, I didn't like it, but it wasn't as if we were married or anything. We didn't even live together.

I handed out the steaming cups and discovered where the marshmallows fitted into the story. The lovely ladies had hidden the sticky sweets in and around their bodies and Tig had adeptly carried out a full stage act of eating them in situ and in front of the large heckling drunken crowd. Gossip had it that he'd gone off with one of the strippers when the party broke up in the early hours, just before three o'clock.

I knew he hadn't because he'd come to me, to my bed, all fired up. But that wasn't the point.

Being as clumsy as I was, I accidentally tripped and spilt the cup of black coffee I handed to Tig when he turned up for work, late. That was the end of our beautiful relationship, such as it was. I'd have liked to give him marshmallows. And nuts. Roasted.

The day I almost met . . .

When you work in the West End you sort of become accustomed to various celebrities and non-celeb wannabes and they would often pass through our revolving doors for one reason or another.

I've walked past a drunken Michael Caine, a skinny Bon Jovi, a bemused Steve Wright, and the newsreader Trevor McDonald who had his head down concentrating on a bundle of papers as he bumped into me while I was in full uniform. I arrested a drummer of a band who had regular top ten hits, arrested C-list celebs for fighting in the street, observed a Hollywood actress who entertained her lover at the Ritz, and had to protect an international singer who was having a hard time in the press. I've investigated the theft of a celebrity's motor when it was found impaled on railings in Mayfair, the stalking of a high-profile comedian turned scriptwriter, and the domestic incidents of a once-alcoholic humorist.

Another time I was on duty in the CID office, a detective in the making, when the DI called me into his office. He had a job that needed doing and he thought DC Sean O'Kane and I would make the right team. This particular job potentially required arresting a big cheese. From Hollywood.

This cheese, an actor, had been secretly having a relationship with a certain high-class model of dusky appearance and foul temper. They'd been together for about eighteen months, very hush-hush but furious gossip and rumour swirled in the paparazzi circles. Nobody had sound evidence. And it's all about the evidence.

The previous night this famous couple had visited Tramp nightclub in the St James area of Mayfair. They'd exited onto the street and were heading for a black limo when a pap pounced, delightedly snapping them in a position that they couldn't possibly deny.

Mr Hollywood didn't like it. He jumped from the limo and grappled the pap to the ground. He wrenched out the film and stamped the expensive camera to smithereens, metal springs and casing crunched into the ground. He may also have given the pap a jab or two, in the style of a raging bull. The pap's face was a mess, smashed tomato style, complete with broken teeth.

DC O'Kane and I had a case of suspected assault and criminal damage. There was also the loss of future earnings for the pap, who took the photo because he could have sold it exclusively and internationally, earning him a fortune. The money and reputation it could have brought would have set him up. It was every photojournalist's dream but it was this pap's nightmare.

The bitter pap had allegedly said to officers the night before, 'She was a worn-out hag anyway.' According to the officer's notes, the pap was like a chattering magpie and not at all complimentary, calling Mr Hollywood an old banger, a worn-out sugar daddy, nothing more than a bare-knuckle thug. Perhaps he was confusing him with a character Mr Hollywood had once played: 'And I don't want him getting away with it! He was like something from the Walsall Mafia. He's cost me big style. I'm selling my story to the News of the Screws so you'd better get to him first, before they do.'

We made our enquiries but nobody would give a statement

until they knew what other witnesses were going to do or say. The CCTV footage was missing, mysteriously wiped. The chauffeur couldn't be traced and the security doormen had suddenly become blind, deaf – and a tad wealthy, some suspected. Then the pap went missing. Did we need to make a report about a missing person? Perhaps he'd been paid off? Handsomely, it was suggested by some.

We had no case. No victim. No evidence. And no arrest.

The DI wasn't happy.

That was the day I learned money doesn't talk: it sometimes buys silence, and everyone has a price.

Marianne St John

Marianne St John was arrested for loitering for the purposes of prostitution. This was a rare occurrence, not because she wasn't a prostitute (she was), but because Marianne was a better kind of street girl who worked as a high-class escort. She was tall, slim, voluptuous, and could be blonde or brunette or auburn, whatever wig or hair dye took her fancy. She was close on fifty but always claimed to be thirty-eight. All the years I knew her, she remained thirty-eight.

Among her clients were Saudi princes and she boasted film stars, politicians and top-ranking officials. Marianne always kept her flat on a council estate in Peckham but it was a base, nothing else. She was forever flying out to far-flung places to be a playboy's plaything, handy for the type of man who preferred to rent rather than buy – his homes, his cars, his boats and his women. Much less maintenance.

It was not unusual for Marianne to spend a fortnight holed up in the penthouse suite of a private apartment block in Mayfair, wined, dined and available to the patron paying for her time, just one of many girls booked for exclusive parties behind closed doors. She would jet off to Dubai before it was a popular playground, or Istanbul, or New York, or wherever her clients wanted her.

She spent three months in Qatar at the beck and call of a very

181

rich man. She said she never had sex with him because he'd had an accident rendering him impotent but he paid her thousands of pounds to be his companion. All he wanted was her attention and affection and he told Marianne he would never find a woman who would give him that with nothing in return and so he was happy to buy it.

She thought it was a sad way to look at life and we both knew he was right.

She had a daughter whose father was allegedly somebody high up in the civil service. Marianne sent her to a prestigious boarding school and whenever her daughter was home from school she would be unavailable for work. She told her daughter she had a good job in the City, working for a billionaire who was happy for her to have the school holidays off.

From time to time Marianne would get bored and go back to her roots. She said it topped up her pin money, gave her a bit of ready cash. She could make a grand a night from cruising Mayfair in her jazzy convertible, snapping up rich pickings from those happy to pay her the right fee.

Marianne was a good girl. We rarely bothered her because she was handy to have on our side. There'd been an armed robbery at a casino and a lone police officer had given chase. One of the gunmen turned on him and the PC was facing double barrels when Marianne cruised by. She saw the standoff and ran the gunman over in her car. She received a judge's commendation and was thereafter immune to arrest from all who knew about it.

It paid off for us to arrest Marianne from time to time, at her request. It kept the other girls off her back and she would pass on tit-bits about various things going down. She wasn't a grass for the sake of being a grass, but like everyone, she had her own code of ethics. If she found out someone had a predilection for paedophilia, she'd happily tip us the nod, irrespective of how well connected they might be.

The night I arrested her she'd asked to be lifted. She had important information she was bursting to tell and the only way to do it was to bring her in officially.

I don't know how she knew, or where she got it from, and we knew better than to ask, but I believed her when she told us there was going to be a bomb planted in a prominent hotel when dignitaries, bureaucrats and others would be attending a sponsored evening event.

This was way out of our league. I'd worked in London long enough to have picked up the pieces from bombings and it's horrific. This was a job for the Bomb Squad.

We contacted the on-call superintendent who arranged for someone to come and collect Marianne.

I don't know the outcome, if there was a bomb or not, but I never heard of a hotel being bombed. Nor did I see her again.

I often wonder what became of Marianne St John.

Phantom of the theatre

There had been a spate of thefts at one of the theatres housing a big West End show. When the main star had something stolen from his dressing room, the powers in charge decided it was time to call the police.

Once it was known the police were involved more staff came forward to say they'd had things stolen. Bizarre things like hairbrushes, a favourite lipstick, a scarf, a fan card, a book.

The cast were a close group as many of them had worked together for years on other shows and didn't want to believe one of their own was stealing. Someone blamed the make-up girl, another the box office staff, and then the ushers were accused. Eventually everyone but the director and the main star was in the frame.

The thefts usually took place during show time, so Barry and I were tasked with spending a couple of nights backstage. We hid up in one of the tiny rooms that smelt of old – old clothes, old brick and old make-up. Once the show started we crept out of our hiding hole to slink against the crumbling walls, looking to catch a thief.

We didn't.

It transpired everyone knew we'd been watching, waiting, so it was no surprise nothing went missing while we were there. We discussed it back at the station and I had an idea. For once our grumpy sergeant agreed. I think perhaps it was because of the high-profile star and the hope of some freebie tickets for the show.

This was going to be a long game. Only one person knew what we were up to. Everyone else thought we'd given up, written if off.

We left it a couple of weeks and sure enough there was another theft. We met the head manager at 4 a.m. with some of the technical guys from the specialist lab based in Lambeth. After a week of close-circuit secret recording we caught our thief.

When we arrested her, she broke down crying. We searched her locker and it was full of everything she'd stolen.

'I only wanted to keep a part of everyone with me,' she sobbed. 'They can have it all back. What's not in my locker, I've got at home.'

She was the chief understudy, everyone's friend and nobody's suspect. Everyone was surprised she was the thief. Nobody wanted to make a statement against her but we had her on camera bang to rights stealing. We had the evidence. What we struggled with were the victims.

The main star, a guy who kept himself to himself, said, 'I think she should be charged to court. It sets an example. You can't catch a thief and let him go.'

The theatre company sacked her.

The CPS ran with the prosecution in the magistrates' court and she pleaded guilty. The magistrates felt sorry for her. She had a lot of mitigation and a lot of support from her ex-colleagues who pleaded for leniency. It helped that she'd undergone psychotherapy for whatever issues she had. She got a bind over because she'd returned all the property and was very sorry. A bind over is the lowest form of punishment a court can give. It meant if she kept out of trouble for the next twelve months it would be forgotten about, no further or future punishment. If she was to be in front of the courts again during that time, she'd be sentenced for these theft offences which could mean a fine, probation, or even prison.

Our sergeant wasn't happy. It had been an expensive operation with what he considered a poor result.

Barry and I managed to get him the main star's autograph.

'Here you are, sarge. From the man himself,' I said, smiling as I handed him an envelope.

He thought it was going to be freebie tickets for the show. I can still hear the roar he gave when he opened it.

Fast train to London

We were supposed to be on the fast train to London, only it wasn't the fast train as it was four o'clock in the morning and it was travelling slower than a stunned slug.

Barry and I had been given the special job of going all the way to Glasgow to collect a prisoner who had been arrested by our Scottish counterparts. When they'd checked him on the system they found he was wanted in London for a minor offence of begging.

It seemed a vast public expense for us to go and bring him back for such a petty crime but it was a matter of justice. He'd failed to turn up at court and so a warrant was issued. You can't disrespect the courts.

Our train was non-stop but we knew non-stop didn't indicate fast. In our case it meant that it travelled through the night, slowly, and didn't stop at any other station.

The prisoner was a wiry chap of fifty-two and he seemed quite happy to be coming with us. He objected to the handcuffs and we decided that given there was no opportunity for him to alight before London we would unleash the beast and take the cuffs off. We sat at a table and placed him in the window seat while Barry and I sat opposite each other in the aisle seats.

Barry was given some dried-up lasagne by the guard when the train restaurant closed. I refused. Barry began to regale us with a sorry tale about the tenant of his flat who'd stolen the three-piece suite because the ceiling had collapsed and then did a runner owing rent money. Scintillating conversation it was not.

I'd had three cups of frothy coffee in an attempt to stay awake but my eyes were sandy and my body weak. It was my twentieth hour of duty and I was tired. I tried to focus on the Celtic knot necklace that our prisoner, Fraser MacKinney, wore but the lines became hazy as my eyelids drooped.

Three hours later, I was woken by someone vigorously shaking my shoulder.

I heard shouting, 'Wake up, wake up. We're here!'

I snapped open my eyes. Barry was snoring like a buzz saw, his mouth as wide open as Jaws. I could see he had black fillings in his wisdom teeth. Yuck. I must be dreaming. I was dreaming. I was kissing someone with a moustache. My eyes closed.

'Miss, you need to wake up. We're at King's Cross. You need to get me to court.'

Ping! I opened my eyes to see MacKinney leaning over the table. MacKinney, who I remembered was our prisoner. He could easily have climbed over his two snoring gaolers and legged it.

I shook Barry awake and tried to retain some dignity.

I turned to MacKinney. 'Thank you. Thanks. Cheers.' It was too much gratitude. 'Sorry but I'm going to have to put the cuffs on you again. Just until the police van comes to pick us up.'

'It's okay, miss. I was glad of the free journey back to be honest. I got mesel' nicked up there 'cos I knew the Met would come an' get me and bring me back to the smoke. You needn't have worried. I was just glad o' the lift.'

'Hmm. Yes. Well. Don't tell anyone will you?' said Barry, slipping him a fiver for some fags. 'We'll get you to court but keep yourself out of trouble. Okay? We'll not be coming back up to Glasgow for you again.'

I think the penalty for losing a prisoner was five days' pay back then, plus a lifetime of mickey taking from every copper who found out. We were more than happy when MacKinney said, 'Cheers, guv'nor. My lips are sealed.'

We got him to court and he was happy to go. A job well done all round. And it was never spoken of again, until today.

Pockets

Trawling the streets looking like lovers but watching for thieves and vagabonds was tedious at times. As the rain lashed down, undeterred tourists flocked to Regent Street, Oxford Street and Soho. Barry and I were drenched and the once-coveted job was now about as shiny as a fake silver charm.

It was times like this that we took to the packed cafés of Hamleys or Burger King or one of the many other places full of people looking to move out of the rain. We were more than justified. Where there are crowds so there are pickpockets.

As we headed for Piccadilly Circus and one of the many tea stops, I spotted him: an older man, dapper, greased-back silver hair, six foot tall and on his own. He was early to mid-sixties and looked like he might be a retired businessman, a husband shopping for his mistress, or maybe looking for something for his grandchildren. He was a man on a mission. I'd seen him loitering outside Hamleys looking through the window, not at it but through it. When I saw him again, looking through but not at the window display of Liberty, I mentioned him to Barry.

'What about that bloke?'

'Yeah, I saw him earlier. Outside Next,' Barry said.

It was the scouring of the inside of the shop, taking in how busy it was, the way he hung back and observed the people. It was the long black Crombie coat, the highly polished black brogues, the way he loitered by-but-not-with a group of tourists. His hesitation, his awareness and his anti-surveillance techniques, looking behind him, doubling back, crossing a busy road at the last minute on the flashing of the green man so that anyone following him would stand out. It was all of that and more.

We tailed him for more than twenty minutes, hanging back, holding hands and feigning chat, trying to hide behind the crowds but keeping him in sight, hoping if he saw us he'd think we were wandering travellers in the melee.

He walked into Marks & Spencer and we lost him.

Barry and I split up. We searched the shop on all levels. Fifteen minutes later we met by the front door escalator. He'd been a dead cert, I was sure of it.

Morose, we made our way to the Oxford Street exit. Out of nowhere he brushed past us and out the door. We were on!

As he walked along the street I noticed a bulge in his coat. It flapped out at the side like a bird's wing. He wasn't carrying a bag and both hands were punched into his side pockets. The coat looked heavier than it had before.

'He's got something, Barry, look!' I said, pointing at the left-hand side of the unbuttoned Crombie.

'Yeah, I noticed too. See what he does next.'

We certainly had enough suspicion to stop and search him but it was better to catch a thief in the act. Or just after. It was a fine line, the prevention and detection of crime. If we waited until he did something and he ran off we might lose him. If we lost him we would have allowed him to commit a crime, but if we stopped him too soon could we prove anything?

The suspect traipsed back down Regent Street. He paused outside the Liberty store once more and raised his hand to his eyes, shielding the reflected light. He didn't enter the shop. He turned and walked on, pondering by a shop selling china and ornaments and other fancy gifts before he walked on again. He strode into Hamleys and wandered around on the first level. He took the escalator downstairs to the café where he meandered around some tables while we hung right back. We watched him take the escalator to the first floor. He didn't buy anything and left the store as empty-handed as he'd entered it.

He could argue he was window-shopping, wasting time, didn't know what he wanted.

We could argue he was looking for a chance, waiting for an opportunity to pick a pocket or two. Or nick a handbag. Or something from a display.

It was nearly four o'clock. Our shift finished at six. We decided to take the plunge. Warrant cards at the ready we stopped him by Waterstones.

'We're undercover police officers, sir,' said Barry, as polite as he ever was. 'We've been following you for over an hour and you've been acting suspiciously. We think you may have stolen items on your person . . .'

'Okay, okay! I knew you were following me. I clocked you in Marksies,' the man said in the best south London drawl.

He gave his name as Terry Archer, his age as sixty-three, and provided an address just south of the river.

We told him our grounds and object of search.

'I know the drill,' Terry Archer said as we moved away from the flow of people and took him to a side street where it was less crowded.

Terry opened up his Crombie and I saw the most fabulous magician's coat I'd ever seen. The coat was full of pockets stitched into the inside, deep pockets from shoulder to hem, each pocket different from the rest and all lined with silver foil. It was a classic shoplifter's trick of the trade. Silver foil carefully adhered to pockets or to the inside of thick sturdy carrier bags deactivates security tags so that electronic alarms at the front doors of shops aren't activated. Anyone found with a silver-lined bag or item of clothing was an instant arrest for going equipped to steal. Thus, we arrested Terry Archer for the offence and Barry cautioned him, to which he made no reply.

When he was searched Terry Archer had a pack of two tea towels in one of the pockets. One tea towel was blue, the other red and both were labelled Marks & Spencer with an £8 price tag.

'What are these?' asked Barry.

'Tea towels, you silly sod,' said Terry Archer.

'You got a receipt?'

'Naw, I nicked 'em,' said Terry, laughing.

And so he was arrested for theft, too.

Terry admitted everything. He was an ex-armed robber and had done plenty of time inside. His criminal record gave him plenty of credentials and was a worthy CV. Terry had promised his son he'd go straight but couldn't help himself. Some habits die hard. He liked the buzz, the thrill, and satisfied himself with petty crime in his retirement.

We charged him to court and knew he'd receive a small fine because his last conviction was more than ten years ago. I had no doubt he'd been active since his last conviction and he'd simply evaded capture. Criminals like Terry considered court fines as a sort of tax.

When Terry found out we would be keeping the coat as evidence, part of the act of committing the crime, and that the court would order its destruction, he was annoyed. He refused to talk to us anymore. The cheeky chappy became the hard man. There was no way we could give him the coat back.

The way things were done had changed, stepped up a gear, just like he had changed, stepping down from armed robber to shoplifter.

Somebody's son

There are some people who turn up time and again. You hope there's a better future for them but you know, like people who do jobs like policing and social work and nursing tend to know, that some can't, or won't, and don't turn their lives around.

Jack Marshall's body lay still, frozen to the ground. A heavy scattering of frost had painted delicate pictures upon him, intricate webs covering his life as he lay there looking angelic, like a statue sculpted in the night.

His clothing offered little protection and when the paramedics thawed his body to move him, I hoped the ripping noise belonged to his frozen T-shirt and tracksuit bottoms, not his skin.

An unopened pack of razors fell from a trouser pocket, a recent theft from the local chemist, the price tag prominent on the packaging. Razors earned good money on the streets, so did bacon rashers, coffee, deodorants, batteries, and expensive sundries usually left hanging on tempting hooks by the entrance/exit of stores.

A bloodied needle rolled from Jack's hand and plopped into a nearby drain, evidence of a recent hit of brown, cheap street heroin.

The paramedics dealt with him in an appropriate way, respectful and considerate, and better than they would have done when he was alive. I knew what they thought, what many thought. Jack Mitchell was no loss to society. It was etched onto their faces like the frost patterns on the dead man's body. They knew like I did, the crime rate would drop over Christmas now a prolific thief was no longer. Statistics would improve all round. Nor would we be called to rescue his battered partner from his violent fists and drunken boorish behaviour.

Pretty Natasha Duggan, drugged up and pregnant, and only sixteen. Perhaps she and her unborn would have a chance, if she chose to take it. What would she call the baby? Jackie for a girl, Jack for a boy, after his dad, because that's what happens when girls have babies by these broken men. They follow the pattern like it's knitted into their soul.

Jack Marshall's mother was heartbroken.

There was a nip in the air when I went to inform Ava Marshall her son had been found dead, half on, half off the pavement on the roadside of Campbell Burn not far from the large sycamore tree on the corner.

I saw her eyes fill and her working woman's hands tremor as she invited me into her council bungalow. Three battered leather chairs, a wonky clutter-topped coffee table and an old-fashioned television sat in the front room. A stack of vinyl records were piled up in the corner and Ava said she'd brought them down from the attic for Jack to see what he could get for them in the secondhand record shop.

A TV magazine ringed with programmes to watch sat on the arm of her chair and I knew she wouldn't see them, not now. *EastEnders. Coronation Street. Holby City.* All the shows that gave her an escape from her own life but which weren't that different from it at all.

I knew the trouble she'd had with Jack over the years. The money he stole from her when he'd called round for his cut on her benefit day, the possessions he'd pawned, the good hidings she'd tried to disguise. I'd met Ava Marshall, and others like her, numerous times.

I noticed the school photograph framed in silver sitting on her mantelpiece. The picture had faded with time and aged with years of stale cigarette smoke. Jack looked about eight, with a cute sparkle in his eye and hope on his face. He had a smudge of dirt on his brow and a crooked parting in his hair. The black and yellow school tie hung wonky and the cheeky grin on his face showed the life he could have lived if he'd made different choices.

'Remember when I brought him home?' I said, looking at the photo, remembering it instantly myself. 'That first time. When he'd wandered off and I found him down by the canal. He was frightened of a caterpillar and all the way home I held his hand and told him how it would turn into a beautiful butterfly.'

Ava Mitchell nodded her head as she wept. Maybe I'd been wrong to remind her of it but I don't think so. I didn't mention the times I'd raided her house early in the morning, looking for Jack and drugs and stolen goods and counterfeit DVDs and more.

I filed away the paperwork, another one to add to the pile of broken lives. I felt a bit sad. Jack might have been a thief, might have been an addict, and he was certainly violent. Those things are difficult to forgive and easy to blame on drugs, society or somebody else, but I remembered that first time.

He had a life once and he was still somebody's son.

Polacc'ed: police car accidents

We were going through a quiet spell. Not much had been happening generally. It either meant the police had been doing a good job at crime prevention or we were doing a lousy one at catching criminals. Either way, it had been an insignificant month. I also mused that it had been a while since I'd had any injuries. Just as you don't say the Q word, quiet, because the minute you do things have a habit of becoming chaotic, I should never have mentioned accidents and a lack thereof.

Barry and I were doing a couple of night duties and we'd been keeping observations on a white saloon car for over two hours. It had travelled through the streets of Soho and Mayfair with us following at a distance in our unmarked police vehicle trying to keep out of sight. We suspected the occupants of delivering drugs to various locations in central London and we now had enough suspicion to stop them. If we started flashing our lights in our unmarked car and indicating for the driver to pull over, they'd think we were mad, or stalkers, so we called for a marked police car. The response was quick. One was on the way to stop the suspect vehicle so that we could search it and the occupants.

By the time the police car arrived, we were travelling along Bayswater Road, trying to hang back. The police driver, PC Steve

Remington, positioned his area car between the bandit car and us. We were all in situ.

The marked police car flashed blue lights and headlights, with a whoop of the sirens, indicating the car in front to stop.

It didn't.

Steve switched on the continuous siren.

The suspect car sped up and we now had a potential pursuit situation with all three cars bombing along Bayswater Road.

The area car hung back, lights flashing. I hoped the suspect car was going to stop though it seemed unlikely as it sharply swung over to the right and then tried to manoeuvre a U-turn in the middle of the road. It pulled wide and collided with barriers on the offside.

'Bloody hell, Ash. That's all we need,' sulked Barry, pulling across the road in front of the now smashed-up suspect car.

I knew Steve Remington wouldn't be pleased. He'd be furious. Although none of our vehicles were involved in the collision, it happened while we were following a suspect car that had crashed. It was a vicinity-only polacc, (accident involving a police car), an accident that didn't involve a police car but happened in front of us or because of our presence. It meant a grumpy night-duty traffic sergeant would have to be called out to the scene along with our sergeant. It also meant a lot of writing. Plus, the vital area car would be out of service for however long it took.

'Oops!' I said.

We approached the crashed car. Barry spoke to the driver, explaining why we wanted him to stop and that we'd be searching the car, all in accordance with PACE, the Police and Criminal Evidence Act.

A black woman with blonde dyed hair sat in the front seat passenger, refusing to move. We ascertained she wasn't injured, just obstinate.

'You have to get out. If you don't we'll have to forcibly remove you,' I said.

She sat as if glued.

'Just get out of the car. Please.'

No response.

The passenger door was damaged and I tugged the handle to open it. It was stuck. I pulled it again, using all my force and both hands. 'You'll have to get out, I can smell petrol,' I said.

She clicked a button on the inside of the door and it sprang open. I poked my head into the car to speak to her and the door flung back. The sharp metal corner of the damaged door smashed directly into my ear. My head exploded. Hot blood dripped down my cheek and fell onto my white T-shirt like fat red teardrops. The sick feeling I get when I hurt myself curdled my stomach, again.

The female suspect pushed the door open and climbed out of the car, pushing past me, oblivious to or uncaring of the blood.

Barry shook his head and called on his radio for a unit to take me to hospital.

'I thought you said it was vicinity-only, no injuries?' said the sergeant.

'I did,' said Barry. 'But that was before Ash got involved.'

How on earth was I going to write up this injury on duty? I was rapidly becoming my own lethal weapon.

That was the night I gave myself a perforated eardrum.

Swinging low

We walked into the party like we were meant to be there. Like we were a cool couple and we'd done this before. And we had. We'd worked together a number of times. But this was our first swingers' party.

It was our brief to be up for swinging, maybe a little nervous because it was our first night and new on the scene. Max was a good-looking guy and we were both single. I guess we were picked for the job as neither of us had partners to be jealous or worried that we'd introduce them to an alternative lifestyle.

The reason for attending the swinging party was to nab a guy suspected of fraud. He'd advertised in the national papers offering jobs abroad working at a new theme park. The unsuspecting potential employees sent him their CV and a cheque for £25 to a PO box. He promised visas and travel arrangements. Everyone had their cheques cashed but there were no jobs. It wasn't a massive amount of money individually but collectively he'd netted thousands. Among the correspondence we found in his postal box was membership to an infamous swingers group.

Our information was that this guy usually attended two out of the three get-togethers that took place every second Wednesday of the month. Members had to phone in on the relevant day to be given details of where and when to attend. Our man hadn't been to the last two gigs, so he was expected at this one. Perfect for us to pick him up.

What to wear for your first swingers' party? I played safe – slim black trousers to emphasise my long legs, heels for added height even though I was naturally five foot nine, and a sort-of transparent white top, which was great for the heady temperatures of Kos but not so hot on a wintry night in November. Perfect for wife swapping, I suspected. Max stood six foot proud with his blond shaggy hair tidied. He was casual in chinos and white shirt open at the collar and he looked good.

We did a recce in a pub near the venue somewhere in southeast London. Anyone not drinking could appear suspicious, a voyeur of the non-sexual type, a journalist or a spy, so the gin and tonics were on the job, full expenses for one night only. We had no idea what Mr X looked like so we were reliant upon the organiser tipping us the wink. The plan was we would approach him double-handed, make him an offer he couldn't refuse, and then lead him outside to be nicked by the waiting team.

Ten o'clock came. It was time to hit the club. We had to be authentic so we held hands in the style of lovers. Our grins of bemusement could easily have been mistaken for a couple in love. Or at least up for something a little different.

Like any other upstairs room in a nightclub, it was compact: dance floor, DJ booth, a small bar, a few chairs and tables and a couple of settees in a quiet corner. The Ladies and Gents were off a short landing behind the DJ.

Coloured roving lights were low and Abba played as the room filled up. I recognised one couple that had been sitting near us in the pub. She looked nervous, near to tears, and kept pulling down her short shift dress. He was antsy, chomping to be away. She didn't want to be there. I wanted to take her away, give her the leaflets for women's help groups and take evidence photographs of the fingertip bruises up her forearm. But it wasn't my remit. I turned away, knowing exactly what was going on there and it wasn't nice.

Max was getting into the vibe and showing off his moves. The guy could dance. I laughed at him and he playfully slapped my arm. I was starting to see what the ladies saw in him. Dangerous territory and I didn't want to go there. I forced him to make me a promise.

'Max, do me a favour?'

He turned to face me, grinning his cheeky boy grin. 'Oh yeah?'

'Don't leave me on my own. Don't go off with anyone.'

'Why? You jealous?' He eyed me up as he took a slurp of gin.

'No! Not that.' I gave him a friendly swipe. 'I mean don't leave me to be picked up. I don't want to get involved in anything I can't handle. I'm not used to this sort of thing and wouldn't know what to say.'

'Neither am I. Just relax, enjoy. Mr X will be here soon so I wouldn't worry.'

We turned back to face the dance floor.

Oh boy! There was a little fat guy in his fifties, a mop of shaggy curls covering his head and matted across his chest, like a hairy bear, complete with a Jason King porn moustache. He was shimmying in the centre of the floor. All but the last button on his Hawaiian shirt was open, gold medallions swaying to a Motown tune. Two tall ladies danced either side of him. Barbies to his Action Man. It wasn't long before they were schmoozing cosily, running manicured fingernails up and down his large exposed belly. I tried hard not to watch with wide-open eyes. I turned to Max and hid my grin in my glass as I swigged the last of my drink. I felt like a schoolgirl peeking into something she shouldn't. I just hoped we weren't expected to join in.

Max and I went to the bar together, neither feeling safe on our own. People dripped into the club in twos, threes and small crowds. There was a lot of handshaking, pats on backs and kissing. I draped my arm across Max's back, feeling protective and insecure. We hadn't discussed the intricacies of how to handle the swingers and this wasn't in the script. I guess we assumed our guy would turn up early and we'd be off without being put to the test.

We stood near the dance floor, bopping away, closer to each other than we'd ever been. I looked to my right and had I not seen it for myself, I wouldn't have believed it. Up against the purple-flocked wall was a granny. Not a young 38-year-old done up like a dog's dinner granny, but a real full-on nana with a grey curly perm, a polyester flowery smock and flat black lace-ups. To her side and facing the wall was a granddad, bald, glasses, braces and sock hold-ups. He had his hand up her dress, exposing her old-fashioned stocking tops. Whatever he was doing, she was enjoying. She was gripping the wall like she might fall off. Or down. He was really giving it some with his left hand. His right hand was hidden. I didn't want to think about what it was doing.

Sitting on a settee facing them was another granny, dressed in similar clothing. She was knitting something blue and avidly watching the performance. She was encouraging them with 'whoop-whoops' and 'go on my son' but I would bet he wasn't her son.

I nearly choked on my gin when Max said, 'You think she's knitting a willy warmer?'

I turned away. I wasn't into voyeurism and I really wished I had missed my evening meal.

Half an hour later Max and I had exhausted small talk. The dance floor was packed. It seemed everything went, nothing was taboo.

I caught a couple giving us the glad eye and I whispered to

Max that we should move. We'd already knocked back a guy who seemed to take a fancy to Max and if we kept making excuses, we'd start to look suspicious.

We bought another drink and I checked with the organiser for any sign of our suspect. Not yet, he confirmed. Max went outside to speak to the other team.

'Another half an hour they said. That's all.'

'Half an hour? Seems a waste to me.' Bravado, the drink talking. 'He might turn up later. We don't want to miss him after all this effort.'

A smooth-looking guy much taller than Max and reeking of expensive aftershave approached us. For some reason our new friend thought Max looked like someone he and his wife had previously entertained. I looked at Max. I hoped not! Then I realised it was a ploy, a tack to get us in with him and his lady. Max hadn't switched on.

They started talking football. A woman joined us. She was petite with a short brown bob and a pretty elfin face. She was wearing a tiny pleated navy skirt, reminiscent of the school netball team, but hers was full and flouncy and flirty. White high heels showed off her slim legs and I could see how a man could be taken in. She wore my favourite perfume and her voice danced with Irish tones. She introduced herself as Aoife, wife of Mr Bonny Prince Charlie who was talking to Max.

Before I could say, 'Hello, goodbye' she'd grabbed Max by the hand and pulled him onto the dance floor. They started dancing to a reggae number.

Max looked over and gave me a little wave.

I shook my head and hoped he wouldn't leave me on my own for too long. I mouthed, 'Stay right there. Don't move.'

I felt the presence of Charlie before I felt his touch on my backside. I shivered and it wasn't in delight. What a creep!

'Ladies, excuse me.' I smiled my best faux smile.

'Oh!' he said. I could see he wasn't used to being turned down.

'Must dash to the loo!' And I left him standing there, hand poised.

I reached the ladies' toilet and in the doorway stood a bloke with a ginger Afro and Elvis Costello glasses. He wore a white T-shirt, which looked like it had come straight out of a packet it was so pristine. On the front it had a peeling transfer of the Bee Gees in psychedelic colours.

'Hi, how you doing?' he said, grinning his gappy teeth at me.

'Hi,' I said, feigning a smile. I moved to the left but he side-stepped me.

He pushed his face close to mine. 'How about it?'

Urgh. *How about what?* I held up a hand. 'Sorry, I'm busy just now. I've arranged to meet someone.'

He pushed the door open for me and grinned. 'Help yourself.'

I thought I'd been saved by quick thinking but soon realised otherwise when I was faced with a sight I could never have imagined. It wasn't pretty. Propped up on a sink with her bottom fully immersed in the basin was a middle-aged woman naked from the waist down. She was being pleasured by two other ladies dressed head to foot in leather. If they were aware of me they didn't show it as they continued on, apparently oblivious to, or unconcerned by, my presence. I rushed into a cubicle and slid the bar across. I slumped down onto the seat, claiming squatter's rights and hiding.

How long could I reasonably be absent? How long could I stay listening but trying not to hear the groans, sighs and grunts on the other side of the door? I groaned myself before realising it might be taken the wrong way. I stood up, straightened my clothing, and touched up my make-up without the use of a mirror. I flushed the toilet even though I hadn't used it, and made my escape, not pausing to wash my hands. I thought it reasonable, under the circumstances.

I walked out of the Ladies without a glance sideways. Up sidled Mr Afro.

'That was quick,' he said.

I mumbled, brain stuttering as I tried to wing it. 'Must dash, catch you later. Bye.' I rushed off leaving him muttering behind me.

I couldn't find Max anywhere. He wasn't where I'd left him on the dance floor. He wasn't by the bar. It was approaching midnight and I needed to find the organiser to check if our guy had turned up. I hoped Max hadn't nabbed him and left me in there on my own. It wasn't safe.

I stepped onto the dance floor and it was like feeding time at the zoo as I dodged groping hands. The DJ squirted choking smoke into the air making it difficult to see and to breathe.

Then I saw him. Max. With his hand up the little lady's skirt. His head was so close to hers that I couldn't see if he was nuzzling her neck or kissing her. I took a deep breath and stepped towards them. I gave him a sharp kick to the shin.

'Ash! Where've you been? Meet Aoife,' he said, a tad under the influence, but I wasn't sure whose – the alcohol or Aoife's.

'Max. We have something to sort out.' I widened my eyes at him, hoping he'd kick into gear.

'In a minute, Ash. I'm busy.' He shrugged me off.

'Max! Now.'

'I'll finish this dance. Be right there.' He buried his head in the bosom of the dear Aoife. 'Come fly with me,' he crooned.

He'd slipped into automatic and forgotten we were on a job. I felt like a nagging wife pulling her husband away from another woman. It didn't feel good.

Max joined me once the song had finished and he'd torn himself away. He gushed, 'She's great. I really like her. They come to these things all the time, her and Charlie. They're only together 'cos of their kids and they don't mind getting off with other people. Keeps them together as a family and they can do as they like without any bother. They've got it sussed, eh?'

'No. Not how it goes, Max. But if it works for them . . .'

'They've invited us back to theirs afterwards. They live in Tottenham.'

'I don't think so, mate. And you'd better not either. We've got a job to do.'

'He hasn't turned up though, has he? Besides, you're single so what's the harm? She's really great, Ash. She put my hand up her skirt. She wasn't wearing any knickers.'

He sniffed his glistening hand.

Urgh! 'Max. You're not thinking straight. You're drunk. It's not on. Right?' I think he really thought it was okay. He was swept up in the experience, the drink, the atmosphere.

'Have a think about it. We can go back, sign off and get up to Tottenham by the time they get home. Their kids aren't there so what do you think?'

'I think Mr X isn't coming tonight and we should leave. Now.'

'I thought you'd be fun. I thought it would be a good laugh. Come on, Ash. Lighten up.'

I pulled him over to the comfy chairs at the back of the club, trying to avoid the gaggle of grannies in the corner who were giving granddads' delight, apart from the one snoring in an armchair with his bottom set of false teeth hanging out.

I got some more drinks and told Max how I'd dodged Aoife's husband, and Mr Afro-guy and the trio in the bathroom. We relaxed, laughed, and he realised Aoife was a fantasy, a no-go. That's how the sergeant found us – giggling in the back seats oblivious to the orgies and shenanigans around us. Sergeant

Bob's eyes were everywhere but we'd become used to it in the three hours we'd been in the club. Three hours? How time flies when you're having fun.

The fraudster didn't turn up. He'd either been tipped off, got cold feet or decided against delights of the flesh that night. I don't know if the Fraud Squad ever caught up with him but I give you my word, I've never felt the need to go swinging again.

I have no idea about Max.

999 hoax calls

Hoax calls take up precious time and can be dangerous. They take up vital resources when the emergency services could be dealing with real crises and saving lives.

Some people call 999 for perverted fun, others because they don't know any better. Police have been called instead of plumbers, ambulances instead of dentists, and the fire brigade for stupid pranks gone wrong. There are the senseless made-up calls, usually kids mucking about, and then there are those that are malicious.

One of our best officers, a family man with young children, was driving a police car one night duty when a 999 call came through. He had the blue lights flashing and sirens blaring. He was driving fast when he crashed at a roundabout. He suffered serious injuries and died two days later in hospital. All because of a hoax call.

Another policeman was on duty one night at a neighbouring station. He attended a 999 call of a report to a car being broken into. It was a hoax made with the intention of the caller to kill the police officer that turned up. The madman shot the PC point blank, hitting him in the chest and killing him outright.

History is littered with similar incidents. It's sometimes difficult not to believe we live in a sick society.

The adrenalin is high when you receive a 999. It's what the people doing the job are trained for. Nobody wants to die a hero but you never ever know what you're going to get when you respond to a 999.

There's a tragi-comedy aspect to the next story, but in reality, they take up time and resources and cost money when we could all be dealing with other things.

A little bit on fire

There was a woman, who I shall call Ruby, who lived on the first floor of a four-storey block of flats. Ruby frequently called the police. She often thought she heard noises, alleged people were breaking in, or she'd claim to have a stalker. She made statements saying she'd witnessed some crime or other, just to get a policeman to her door. They were all false allegations and made-up crimes.

She admitted she liked a man in uniform and I think one or two had succumbed over the years. Or perhaps that's malicious rumour and supposition. Ruby wasn't unattractive. She had a nice figure, a cheeky grin and a deep cleavage that many would consider a feature. When she wasn't drunk and you met her in the street, she'd stop and smile and be very cheery. It was only late at night, when she was lost and lonely in drink that she called 999. Ruby was married but her husband worked away on the rigs, which meant she was home alone for weeks at a time. We always knew when her old man was away because the calls would be frequent.

One night our inspector said, 'Enough!'

Just after midnight Ruby called 999 reporting someone breaking into the empty flat above hers.

The inspector heard the message over the radio and called me.

'Ash, I want you to go. Tell her from me, any more false calls and she's going to get herself lifted.'

I took Tim, one of the probationers. His eyes popped out as Ruby answered her door dressed in black stockings and suspenders, a pink baby doll nightie, and drenched in sickly perfume and sour alcohol.

Her mouth dropped into a sulk as she looked at me. She reached out a hand to stroke Tim's arm.

I batted her away from my colleague.

'Ruby, we've been upstairs to check the empty flat. There's nobody there. You've got to stop calling the police. You're going to get yourself into trouble.'

'What did they send you for? They know I always want a man,' she pouted.

'Join a dating agency then but stop calling us. The inspector said if you call again, I'll have to arrest you so please stop it. We haven't got time to keep turning up here on false calls and I'm sure the last thing you want is to spend a night in a cold police cell.'

'You could always leave this one here for me.' She pointed a red nail at Tim, almost touching his nose.

He stepped back, a tad bewildered. I thought he was going to run.

'Enough, Ruby. This is your last warning. Okay?' I said.

She turned and slammed the door.

We didn't hear from her for months and then one night duty as I was making the tea, again, a 999 call came out. A report of a fire with persons trapped. These calls are always horrible. I particularly hated fires, having been in one as a child. They filled me with dread.

I was halfway to the address before it registered it was Ruby's flat. I hoped it wasn't a hoax. I hoped it *was* a hoax. I wouldn't wish anything bad on her.

Two fire tenders were there when we arrived and a dozen firemen all suited up and ready to fight the flames. Ruby stood on the doorstep, wobbling drunk and half-naked in her underwear. A boob was almost hanging out and I wanted to rush over and cover her up.

A couple of the firemen were laughing. The officer in charge wasn't impressed. This call was the latest in a long line of false calls made to them by Ruby.

My warning of arrest had stopped her calling the police but instead she'd turned her affection to the London Fire Brigade.

Ruby drunkenly leant against her doorframe. 'Show me your tools, boys. You got a big hose for me?'

The officer in charge said, 'Last week she called to say a pussy was stuck. Before that she said her flue was alight. Always some innuendo. But this is serious. Persons trapped is high priority.' He was furious.

'I know. She'll have to come in,' I said. I edged my way to her front door.

Ruby saw me. 'You! What the fuck do you want? I called the fire bobbies, not the polis.'

'You phoned 999 to say there was a fire with people trapped inside a burning building. It's not on, Ruby. You'll have to be arrested this time. I did warn you. Let's get you some clothes on. You'll have to come with me.'

'But I'm still a little bit on fire,' she said, giving me a sulky look.

I arrested and cautioned her and did feel a bit sorry for her. She was lonely and drink made her behave badly.

She was really remorseful once she'd sobered up. She was an intelligent woman who couldn't have children and her husband worked away. She'd given up work after her last miscarriage years earlier and she said she didn't have the confidence to try and find a job. She was manic-depressive and verging on alcoholic. Everyone has a background story and this was hers. Mitigating tragedy.

Ruby went to court and pleaded guilty. She had no choice. She'd made more than fifty false calls to the police and the fire brigade in the past year. We hadn't realised there were so many until we pulled the information together. She was given a hefty fine and agreed to have counselling and to seek help for her drinking. It was a chance to rebuild her life and I hope she took it.

Night-duty eyes

You have to do a lot of odd shifts when working undercover, most of it during the late evening and night, for reasons you'd best ask nocturnal criminals. I did a heck of a lot of night work and although I loved night duty, it batters the body somewhat. I still sit up in the middle of the night wondering what time it is and if I should be at work yet.

Researchers have done many studies regarding shift workers and the effects of working during the night. There are suggestions that it increases the risk of cancer, causes a lack of melatonin, disrupts bodily functions and is generally bad for your health. That's all well and good but society needs night-duty workers in a variety of professions and someone has to do it.

There's this phenomenon we called 'night-duty eyes'. I'm sure all night workers will know of it. It usually occurs in the latter half of the night shift, or on the way home.

You see things. Strange things. Figments and filaments of the imagination. Things that flit in front of your eyes that aren't really there. Ghosts, maybe. Shadows. Odd stuff. Flashbacks. Perhaps it's the brain trying to make sense of things, filtering out the rubbish and fooling you. Perhaps they are a form of hallucination but you'd never get a copper confessing to having one of those.

I remember a sergeant driving his car on his way home from night duty. He came running into the police station to say he'd seen a woman in a nightdress by the side of the road, near to the flyover. The area was searched thoroughly. There was nobody reported missing or any other call of distress regarding this lady. She wasn't found. It was put down to night-duty eyes, though he was adamant.

Rolled-up pieces of carpet take on the form of dead bodies, animals run out in front of you only to disappear again, and shadows take on the appearance and movements of deadly beasts.

I was on my fifth night of undercover obs, working with a dour guy called Vic. We were keeping watch on a factory that made exclusive clothes for top designers as we'd received a tip-off it was going to be burgled. Another team was watching from the rear. Next to the factory sat a cemetery. It had high iron gates and large stone pillars at the entrance.

After a couple of hours of boredom and silence, my eyes were drawn to movements by the graveyard. I sat up in the passenger seat of our unmarked police car and pointed to the gates of the cemetery. 'Vic! Vic. There they are.'

'Who?' he mumbled. 'I can't see anyone.'

'There, over there!' I pointed to the cemetery. 'Look. Sitting on top of the pillars, a guy sitting on each one.'

'What are you on about?' he said, sitting up and peering over the steering wheel.

'There. Two guys. By the cemetery gates.'

'No one's there. I'm the one wearing glasses. You want to try 'em?' he said.

'Don't look at me as if I'm mad. There's two guys and they're talking to each other. One's wearing a white T-shirt, the other a black jacket,' I insisted.

'A T-shirt! In this weather? I'm telling you, there's no one there. You're seeing things.'

We were each as persistent as the other.

'I'll show you,' Vic said. He started the car and drove with the lights off.

'Don't do that, they'll leg it,' I said.

'Yes. Because there's nobody there.'

I kept my eyes on the two men as Vic drove, inching forwards to make his point.

I blinked. Blinked again. I rubbed my eyes. There wasn't anybody there. No one at all. Of course I had to apologise. 'Sorry,' I said sheepishly. 'Night-duty eyes.' I'd been so sure two guys had been sitting there, chatting. I seriously wondered if I was going mad. Or if they be ghosts . . .

Luckily for me, Vic wasn't one for jokes or leg pulling and he didn't say anything to anyone. I'd have heard about it if he had.

And I'm still not convinced there wasn't a man sat on each plinth . . .

On the job

Walking around the police station it's easy to forget some people don't know who you are when you're in plain clothes. Why should they unless you've worked with them before and they know you?

I suppose I shouldn't blame him, that sergeant; it wasn't his fault, but it does prove the point about stereotype and gender perception. I found it all rather funny.

Barry and I had nicked a guy for deception. He'd been doing a bit of credit card fraud and had run up bills amounting to over twenty thousand pounds when we collated all the evidence. His description had been circulated across All Stations (an all stations bulletin) and all squads had his photograph.

We were vigilant in tracking him down. We knew he preferred the upmarket kind of store, such as Burberry, Fortnum & Mason and Austin Reed. Our target was to find him and we did, catching him in the act when he attempted to buy a fancy Montblanc fountain pen at a price of £215, cheap in the sale.

He gave his name as Anton Ponsonby. It was the name embossed on one of the cards in his wallet. He had other cards in the name of Jeremy Fitzharbour and Bartholomew Woods and Barney Fairweather. He was nattily dressed, looked the part of well-to-do gentleman, with his highly polished black shoes, jeans with a good cut, white Charles Tyrwhitt shirt, open at the neck and with double cuffs, complete with a grey sleek overcoat. I suppose he was good-looking with his smooth chiselled face, brooding eyes and a scar that cut deep into an eyebrow. He spoke well and was charming, though he didn't fool me like he fooled the shop assistants. I imagined him the anti-hero in the very best Jill Mansell novel.

When we took him to the station to be booked in, both custody sergeants were busy so we took a seat on the bench along the back wall of the charge room to wait our turn. It was going to take some time to get our Clark Gable look-alike booked in so Barry went off to make some enquiries with the credit card companies while I sat with him.

There is never a need to be unpleasant to people you arrest, unless they are violent or abusive, in which case you restrain and ignore them. I chatted with our suspect about minutiae, avoiding the subject of his arrest. We were still chit-chatting when one of the sergeants looked at my prisoner and beckoned him forth.

'Bring her over,' the sergeant said.

We both remained seated.

'Come on. I'm ready now. I can get her booked in,' he said, looking at us both.

I looked at the guy next to me. I looked at the sergeant. I pointed to my chest. 'You think I'm the prisoner?'

'Clark Gable' took my arm and pulled me up. He was laughing, a right royal hee-haw belly laugh. 'Come on then. Let's be having you.'

I shrugged him off, not sure whether to laugh or fall to the floor. I pulled out my warrant card from my jeans' back pocket and placed it in front of the sergeant.

'Ash Cameron, Crime Squad. We've been doing surveillance looking for this man.' I pointed at our prisoner. 'We caught him using a stolen credit card so I arrested and cautioned him for deception and he made no reply. He has other credit cards in different names on his person, sarge.'

Sarge had the shame to blush. Our prisoner found it extremely funny. So did the second custody sergeant who had been quietly chuckling away, keeping schtum.

It was only when Barry and I were writing up our notes prior to interviewing Clark Gable that Barry told me the sergeant had thought I was a tom.

Charming. Not. But I never did let on that I thought it was kind of funny.

Dead ringer

I've never been into fast cars or fast driving. I drive because it's a necessity and it gets me places. If I have a choice, I'll always let someone else do it.

For a few years my journey to work was long. It was almost thirty miles from my house, a sixty-mile round trip. I could drive it in thirty-five to forty minutes if I was on an early morning shift or late evening. In rush hour it could take two hours or more. Otherwise, I could go to the nearest tube station and have an hour on the District line. That was okay because starting at the end of the line I always got a seat on the way in. Coming home I was with the commuters vying for a vacant space and dodging wandering hands and bad breath until at least Dagenham.

Our area commander arranged for us to have the use of the bottom level of an NCP car park at cheap rates, the same car park where Simon Cowell had apparently run his promotions office in the basement during that era. I never saw him. But if I did, I wouldn't have known him back then. It's reported he used to dress up in animal suits for his day job in promotions. Who would have known that the badger I'd dodged would be so rich and famous today?

It was a great perk for those of us living beyond the tube line because we were given priority passes for the car park. The bosses agreed to it because if we did overtime or worked a late-late shift there was no way of getting home once the tubes shut down. Night-duty officers would have had to give a lift to all those officers who couldn't get home and they usually lived at any of the compass points from central London. Doing transport duty took valuable police officers off the streets. I once spent a whole night duty driving around the M25 dropping people home. When I got back to the station round 4.30 a.m., I had cells full of prisoners to deal with. Hence the great perk of car parking.

My own car was an Astra. It was serviceable, comfortable and it had a good radio. Astras were used as police cars too, but instead of a stripe and a blue light, mine was plain silver. I bought it cheap from a garage near to where some friends lived up North. A reputable garage, apparently.

I'd had it for about eight months when there was a hefty rap on my front door. I was about to leave for work, my hair almost dry, make-up half on, when I answered the persistent ringing doorbell to a pair of plain-clothed officers from the National Crime Squad, based in Manchester.

'Ash Cameron?' the taller of the two asked.

'Yes?' I was confused. Why would they be at my front door?

The shorter one turned to his colleague and said, 'Told you it was a woman.' He turned back to me and said, 'Is this your car?' pointing to my Astra on the drive.

'Yes. It's a fair assumption. Is there a problem?'

'There is. Can we come in?'

I knew enough to let them in and make them tea. 'What's it about? I'm in the job. I work undercover. For the Met.'

Really?' said the one who introduced himself as DS Alastair Laing. 'We weren't aware of that.'

I don't suppose there was any reason why they would know.

There was no database that listed police officers and where they lived and what their cars were. Unless I was deep undercover, involved in something a bit murky and had a different identity, but I wasn't doing anything like that. I showed them my warrant card and gave them the details of my boss so they could verify me.

'I'm just about to leave for work for a twelve till eight shift and I've got to get into central London. If I don't leave soon, I'll be late,' I said.

'I suggest you ring your boss then, love,' said the DS.

I hate being called 'love', so patronising, especially from people you don't know, but lots of people use it. 'Yeah. I'll give him a ring. Do you have any ID? Just so I can let my sergeant know when I ring him.'

It was my turn to write down their details: DS Laing and DC Street. I made the call and I was good for a couple of hours.

They showed me a PNC printout which held the details of my car. I was no longer the registered keeper. It was registered to some guy I'd never heard of who lived in Sunderland. They asked for every detail of where and when I'd bought the car, how much I'd paid, how I paid; they asked for my insurance documents and any work I'd had done on the car. They then they asked if I'd ever had an accident in it.

'Don't panic, love. We think you have the original motor. There's another silver Astra running around with your reg plate on it. We wouldn't normally tell you this but as you're job too . . . it was used in an armed robbery in Salford a few weeks ago. We've been to see the bloke in Sunderland and impounded his car. We just need to check out yours. The chassis and engine numbers and that. We'll take a statement and see what we can do for you but the boss might want us to bring it in. His call. All right?'

All right? What choice did I have? My car was a suspected ringer. I didn't like it at all but what could I do?

It all checked out okay and they didn't take the car but they did warn me there was a marker on the computer. 'Listen love, just to warn you, you might get a pull if anyone did a PNC check on your motor. Oh, and don't sell it,' DS Laing warned. 'It might take us a bit of time to sort it all out. We'll be in touch.'

Every time I took a trip, I was anxious. I tried to use the tube or the train as much as I could. I decided against visiting faraway friends and relatives on my days off, just as a precaution. I felt like I might be a criminal, though knew I wasn't. And I didn't fancy trying to prove it all to a Norfolk traffic cop or a Scouse detective.

A couple of months later I received a letter to say the National Crime Squad were allowing me to keep the car and the marker had been taken off the PNC. However, I then had the job of sorting it all out with the DVLA and trying to change the registered keeper details back into my name.

The lesson I learned was to never again buy a car from that poky little garage on the corner where my friends used to live. I also learned that anyone can unwittingly become a suspect and it didn't feel good being on the other side, even though I knew I had done nothing wrong. Of course, I was Ash-who-doubled-as-an-armed-blagger to the lads at work for a little while. It was a talking point and afterwards we had a good laugh. Trust me to pick up a ringer! I hated bloody driving anyway.

And there is nothing like being on the other side for a touch of reality and empathy to kick in.

Perks

Some police departments have contracts with vehicle hire companies and from time to time we would use these rental cars for special assignments. We were authorised to use our own vehicles for things like making enquiries, taking statements and general running around, but our personal cars became known and we'd stand out as much as if we'd had POLICE written across the doors and a blue light flashing. If we had to travel to far-flung places such as Milton Keynes or Nottingham, it was cheaper to use a hire car than to pay us mileage to use our own vehicles. I've used plenty of hire cars because lots of our enquiries took us all over the UK.

I know some squads bought cheap old bangers when they needed to dumb it down, to meld in, and then they sold them off for scrap once they were finished with, but I never had an under-cover job that warranted that.

I was due to have a hire car delivered to me at home one evening for a job which required a lot of mileage and would take us some-where in middle England.

By nine o'clock at night it still hadn't arrived at my home address and I started to get impatient, thinking they'd forgotten me. I was worried the five o'clock early start would have to be postponed and was wondering if it was too late to phone the sergeant at home.

I was in the kitchen making a cuppa when Kenny shouted from the living room. 'Ash, I think your car's here!'

'At last!' I stomped through to the lounge and pulled the curtains aside. 'Don't be daft,' I sighed. 'That's not our car.'

'Well the guy who was driving it is now walking up our path,' said Kenny.

'It won't be for us. You see to him, I'll finish off making the coffee.' Honestly, did he really think the job would pay for a five series top-of-the-range white glossy BMW?

I heard the guy at the door say, 'Ash Cameron? Well she'll have to sign for it. Has to be the person on my log, sorry.'

I dropped the teaspoon and walked up the hall to have another look. I pointed at the car parked on the street. I was open-mouthed. 'That? They've given us that?'

'Err . . . yeah. Is there a problem? It's the only car we had left that was any good and 'cos it's the police contract, well, we knew you'd want something decent. I'll take it back if you like but my guv'nor said to bring it anyway. Your boss usually asks for a good motor.'

'Really? No, no! It's fine. But . . . will it cost much more?' I could see our department budget disappearing along with my head if they were going to charge us the usual daily rate for a top-class BMW.

'No. Same price. No extra cost. Just sign at the bottom there, cheers.'

I wasn't going to argue. I signed the form.

When I went to collect Jas the following morning she did a double take and asked the same questions I had. Her fingers glided over the smooth white leather seats as she slipped inside the car.

'It's only got fifty-five miles on the clock,' I grinned. 'You can drive it back if you like.'

It wouldn't have been practical for some jobs to use a car like that as we would stand out like a beacon and certainly attract attention, but for this one we were gathering intelligence and information and taking statements concerning a paedophile ring, so it was fine. It wasn't often we got perks and it's the one and only time I've ever driven a car like that.

Unlike my mate Barry who once got a Porsche!

Lucky ladders

You have the best sleeps after a hard night's work. Falling into bed, wrapping a soft quilt around you while the world is waking up is delightfully delicious. It never took long for sleep to take me after a night duty. I could rest without fear of missing the alarm and knew I'd never sleep in.

It was in the middle of summer during one of my deep sleeps that I became aware of a tinkling sound, like tapping on glass, of windows rattling. Panic brought me up sharp, the flight or fight syndrome that many emergency workers hone to perfection. Someone was trying to break in!

I didn't know what time it was, or even where I was. I jumped up out of bed, groggy and hungover, not from drink but from not enough sleep. The rattling was insistent and urgent, and my fuzzy brain translated it into imminent invasion.

I was back on obs, lying in wait for a team of burglars.

I heard myself yell, 'Go, go go!'

I grabbed the curtains. Flung them apart.

I stood at the bedroom window, naked, facing our very attractive French window cleaner.

He wore a look of surprise.

I wore nothing.

My head and my heart pounded. I swept the curtain closed, almost bringing down the rail. I was mortified with embarrassment, my brain confused, my body adrenalised. I don't know who was more traumatised, me or the window cleaner.

It took him a few weeks to knock for his money.

I could only hope nobody reported me for flashing.

Downfall

I had a long weekend off so I returned to my hometown to see a friend, Jackie, who'd just had a baby. We went for a quiet night out, just the two of us. It was a pleasant evening. She wasn't drinking and I wasn't drunk. It was nearing midnight when we went looking for a taxi. We didn't find one but we did find an unconscious girl. She had collapsed in the melee of the town centre and was slumped against the wall of the library.

I bent to check for a pulse. Two youths approached and asked what I was doing.

'I think she's fainted. I'm not sure. Could you call an ambulance?' I asked.

'What the fuck's it got to do with you, like?' leered the one eating chips from a wrapper.

This wasn't going very well.

'I'm an off-duty police officer,' I said, turning back to the girl on the floor.

Thwack! The other guy thumped me, hard, across the back of my head. I fell forward and onto the unconscious girl. I tried to stand, one hand against the pebble-dashed wall that prickled my palm.

The guy eating flung his flaccid, fatty chips into my face. I stumbled and fell backwards over the legs of the girl. Then they started the kicking.

A police patrol car cruised by, in no hurry to stop. My frantic friend flagged them down.

'Do you really need the aggravation?' they said as they let the youths leave. 'Anyway, she's just a junkie. Do you know her?'

Of course I didn't know her.

'No. Never seen her before. But she's unconscious and needs some help. I tried to help and these guys attacked us.' I could have wept but didn't want to cry.

'Really? It's your word against theirs, ladies. And your friend who called us, well, she's just had a baby. Do you need that hassle?'

'Hassle?' I asked, confused.

'Well, you know, you've been drinking.'

'Drinking? My friend is breast-feeding. She wasn't drinking. And I've only had two halves of lager and lime. Not even in a pint glass.' I don't know what difference that made but I was back home, back North where women usually drank pints along with their men.

Neither of the lads had a mark on them. They wouldn't have because nobody touched them. I was covered in scuffs and cuts and bruises. I didn't understand. Since when did having a baby mean that you couldn't be a credible witness? If every witness or victim was dismissed because they'd imbibed a small amount of alcohol we'd have hardly any cases in court at all.

'I don't get it. They attacked me because I tried to help her,' I protested.

'Just forget it, love. It's Friday night.' The officer snapped his notebook shut.

'But I'm in the Met!' I protested.

'The Met? Why didn't you say? That makes it crystal clear. Forget it.' The officer walked off and climbed back into his police car.

The following morning, after I'd been to hospital, I went to the police station. I had an injury to my neck and back and the doctor had given me a padded collar, which he said I had to wear for at least five days. I had a bruise the size of a football on my back and a large bruise to my right calf.

The desk sergeant took a report. He said, 'There's no CCTV covering there. It will be difficult to trace the youths. There's no record of a girl fitting the description having been taken to hospital or arrested and in custody.'

I could describe the officers but I knew it was doubtful they'd made a pocket-book entry, so it would be difficult to track them down. The old-fashioned desk sergeant said the best advice he could give was that I was better off forgetting the incident.

I returned to London in a stiff padded collar and wore the black and blue bruises like unwanted badges. It was none of my concern. I should have learned not to get involved in things off duty, but I could never walk away from someone who needed help.

Ailsa MacPhee

Barry and I had a tip-off about a drug deal going down. We made our way to an underground car park halfway between Mayfair and Soho. It made all the difference in the world, that distance between Mayfair and Soho, where the aroma of fancy garlic mingles with dirty drains.

We did a reconnaissance to find the best vantage point. The car park was expensive, five pounds for half an hour, one of those places filled with Jaguars, Rolls-Royces, BMWs and eclectic sporty numbers. I dread to think what they would cost today.

A silver soft-topped BMW with a private registration was parked in the basement and as we approached, a young girl climbed out of the front passenger seat. It was obvious to me what she'd been up to as she wrapped her light raincoat around her thin body and pocketed something. Money. Maybe a used condom. Probably both.

I bent down to take a look at the other person in the car. He was much older than her, grey hair, smart suit. He leant back in the driver's seat and pulled up his fly.

She was in a hurry, a flurry of litter swirling around her feet as she rushed off.

I followed her, warrant card ready.

'Leave it!' Barry whispered.

He was interested in burglars and drug dealing and hard knocks, but this girl looked young. Too young. Especially too young for prostitution.

I followed her onto the street. When I was close enough I reached out and touched her shoulder.

She spun round, tottering on heels that were too high.

I flashed my warrant card. 'Who's the guy in the car?'

'He's someone I know . . . a family friend . . . sort of . . .'

I knew she was lying. 'Please open your coat.' I wanted to see if she was dressed for the job. I hoped I was wrong.

She refused. 'Please. Please don't do this,' she begged. 'Just let me go.' Her dwarf-rabbit eyes pleaded with me.

We were jostled by a group of suits leaving a restaurant. One of them eyed her up. I scowled at him and grabbed her arm. I took her into a side street.

She threw three £20 notes onto the pavement. 'There! There you go! Is that enough for ye?' She broke down in tears, her little red face crumpled with its too-old-for-her make-up smeared across her cheeks.

I had no option but to take her in, not under arrest but under 'place of safety'. She was fourteen and like so many others on the street she was far too old for one far too young.

Nobody had bothered to report her missing. Nobody cared. But there were plenty of punters ready to pick her up off the meat rack of Shaftesbury Avenue, or the false-economy pavements of Shepherd Market where she loitered outside the back doors of famous restaurants waiting for passing punters and any scraps the kitchen-hand threw her way.

While we waited for social services to come she told me the typical story, one I'd heard time and again. She'd been abused by her stepfather and various 'uncles' and it was a very sad life.

'I had to keep house in a home my mother long left. I dunnae where she went when she disappeared. I just had to look after them, cook an' clean an' a' tha' . . .' She didn't need to tell me explicitly what the a' tha' meant. It was in her eyes like it always was with kids like her.

As we talked she doodled on the back of blank statement forms. She drew faces of men. She was good at drawing, with an attention to detail that captured something only someone who'd been to those dark places could replicate. She told me about selling her soul to the devils who would pay and about how it was the only thing she had to trade. Her stories were hard and she was practical. It was the only thing she knew to do to survive. She had a look in her eyes that glinted fear and danger. I saw her as vulnerable and feisty, her elfin face framed by dark hair in desperate need of a wash. She also had a finger missing on her left hand, the result of a bad accident, and that's all she would say as her eyes filled with tears and bad memories.

I changed the subject and talked about how creative she was and what a marvellous gift she had. I wanted to make her feel better.

My sergeant said it wasn't my job to deal with runaways. Or prostitutes. If I wasn't interested in his crime operations, he didn't appreciate me sorting out waifs and strays.

'There's real criminals to be caught, Ash,' he warned. 'Juvenile bureau might suit you better.'

Social services emergency duty team found someone to come and take my girl away from the streets with lights bright and full of fake promise, different from the place it was during office hours when street people would scurry and hide like the rats that danced only in the dark.

Over the weeks and months, I wondered how she was, where she was, what she was doing. I couldn't forget that wee lassie from a place called Leuchars in Scotland. She had touched something deep down inside.

And then from nowhere she turned up. I didn't instantly recognise her. The straight dark hair in need of a wash and pushed back with an Alice band had long gone. It was now short, blonde and spiky. Her face was changed, older somehow. And she had a tattoo on her neck, two rough diamonds intertwined. It looked homemade. She didn't speak. I had to take her fingerprints for formal identification. I had to search her. Her purse was empty of money but contained two things: a national insurance card and a scrap of paper with my name and phone number on it. I wondered what it would have taken for her to call. I wondered if she had considered it. Whatever, in the end, she hadn't. I felt sad. I didn't have to take her prints to confirm her identity. I knew it was definitely her. I recognised the little dark dwarf-rabbit eyes filled with hopelessness. And I noticed the missing finger. That's when she spoke to me the loudest. A dead body on a slab whose fingerprints I had to take.

It's a rotten job sometimes, working the streets of London. Especially when you're dealing in lost souls and learning you can't save them all. I'll never forget her, little Ailsa MacPhee, from Leuchars, in Scotland somewhere.

A quick buck

It was one of those Saturday afternoons that started off badly. A third of our squad had taken leave or called in sick. Others had been sent to do football duty. In uniform. That left six of us, including the sergeant who decided he had other things to do. Matt and Gary had prisoners from the night before to deal with. Max had to go to West London to take a statement for a pending court case. That left Barry and I.

We grumbled as we read the bulletins in the Local Intelligence Office (previously known as the Collator's office). It was full of indexes of information and files full of dubious people and their proclivities. Photographs of suspects and convicts adorned the walls.

'There's been another robbery at a bureau de change. This time in Tottenham Court Road,' said Barry, reading from the log.

'Getting closer. Isn't that five now? What's the script?' I asked.

Barry read on. 'Male, IC1 [the identity code for ethnicity, in this case a white person], eighteen to twenty-five, five foot six, holds up the change kiosk and threatens the cashier with a snub-nosed pistol, demands sterling and dollars only. Wears a cowboy-style neckerchief. Bloody hell!' He paused. 'Can you believe it? He snapped up six grand yesterday! It was twenty to six so plenty of people were about. No CCTV but there's a grainy pic from when he did the one at King's Cross.'

I looked at the black and white image. 'Rich pickings, eh? No accomplice?'

'No mention of one. Seems like a one-man bandit.'

'As opposed to a one-arm bandit,' I chuckled. I don't think Barry found it very funny.

'Hard to pick out of a crowd though,' I said, making a note of the suspect's description in my pocket book. 'What else?'

'Usual. Three handbags stolen, a van-dragging in Old Bond Street, half a dozen purses and wallets lifted. Dodgy notes going around Oxford Street. Bad Fatacc in Baker Street. A making off without payment in Mayfair. And some dodgy drugs going around Soho. Nothing much in the way of any suspect info for any of it really.'

We went to book out a radio only to discover there weren't any. We checked the front office and various other places where we might find one lying around. Nothing. All we had were pagers. We could be contacted but we couldn't contact anyone.

With more wittering and bemoaning we set off into the crowds. Barry was grumpy. I put it down to tiredness because we'd finished late the previous night. 'I hope we don't have to call for any assistance,' he moaned. 'Pointless! And I don't want to be late tonight. I've got plans.'

I should have known then. If anything was going to go awry it would always be when you least wanted or needed it. Again, like the Q word, you just don't mention 'plans'.

We spent a couple of hours trawling Regent Street and other tourist-packed avenues. Around five o'clock we considered calling time but Oxford Circus was teeming with people, like someone had pulled a plug and everyone had flooded in. We decided to give it another half an hour and loitered at the top of Argyll Street, watching, looking out for faces, known criminals, any suspicious activity.

We'd been standing there for only two or three minutes when Barry nudged me in the midriff.

'Oof! Five minutes since you last asked,' I said. 'Five past five.'

He turned to stand in front of me, an inch from my face. His voice was an octave higher than usual. 'Behind me. The doorway next to the bureau de change. It's him.'

I glanced in the opposite direction and then did a casual sweep above head level so that I wouldn't catch anyone's eye, should they be looking. I draped an arm around Barry's neck and rested my head on his shoulder. I looked at the guy stood in the doorway. The fuzzy photocopied picture flashed in front of me. It was him. He was more like five foot ten, stocky with short cropped fair hair, but it was him. The red and white bandana around his neck confirmed it.

'Sure looks like it, buddy,' I said. 'How should we do this?'

'Bit difficult without a bloody radio. What's he doing?'

'Just standing there. Looking around, biding his time.'

I felt the adrenalin hit. My head pounded, both eyes hurt behind the eyeballs, my stomach and chest fluttered, the soles of my feet tingled. It's times like this, you're most alive.

'Can you see a gun?' asked Barry.

'Nope. He's got his arms crossed. Maybe it's in his pocket.' He wore a casual jacket over a T-shirt and jeans. I kept my eyes down but could see him in my peripheral vision. 'There's one customer at the change kiosk, an Asian guy. When it's empty, he'll be in. He's building up. Keeps going on tiptoes, his eyes everywhere. He's antsy.'

'You go to the tube station, Ash. Get the staff to call 999. I'll keep watching but if he goes for it, I'll have to have him. Hurry up.'

I didn't want to leave but knew we needed help and fast. Oxford Circus tube station was a few feet away. This was no time to politely ask for a parting of the crowds. As soon as I knew I was out of sight, I ran. I ran for my life, down the tube station steps and onto the concourse. I couldn't see anyone. No staff were loitering like they usually did. None waited at the top of the escalators. I ran to the ticket office and barged my way through irate tourists and shoppers. I held my warrant card up and shouted at the person behind the screen. 'Please phone 999. There's a robbery about to take place by the bureau de change in Argyll Street. Quick. He's got a gun!'

The startled man behind the counter looked at me and stared. And kept staring.

'I'm a police officer. Please ring 999. There's a robbery taking place right now! Argyll Street.'

I spun round and lost my bearings. In my panic I couldn't remember which exit I needed. I ran to each one twice before I took a chance. I had to get back onto the street. I took the stairs two at a time, pushing people out of my way. My heart beat in the back of my throat.

I was relieved to breathe the sharp air on the right side of Oxford Street. I couldn't, didn't, pause. I only hoped the ticket man had phoned the police. My eyes flicked over the confusion of heads in front of me as I searched for Barry. I couldn't see him.

Then I did.

He was standing next to the suspect, ignoring him, nonchalant, as if waiting for someone. At that moment the customer in the kiosk walked off.

The bandana went up. The suspect reached into his right-hand jacket pocket. He left the doorway and walked into the tiny bureau de change.

Barry followed. He hadn't seen me. I heard sirens in the distance and prayed they were coming our way. I rushed over and gently nudged Barry in the back as I took my place beside him.

The suspect pulled out a small silver handgun.

'Fuck!' I think Barry might have said it. Or maybe it was me, in my head. Or perhaps out loud.

Barry grabbed the gun arm, swinging it around and up the back of the suspect, and fell forward, pressing the suspect against the counter. I tried to sweep the legs from under the gunman and we all fell to the ground in a kerfuffle. It really wasn't anything like you see on the telly. Barry and I sat on top of bandana man and we both scrabbled to get the gun out of his hand, fearing he might pull the trigger, accidentally or otherwise.

One or both of us shouted, 'Weapon! Weapon!'

Because of the position of his arm, the gun fingers were twisted and unfortunately, they couldn't bend to release the weapon, not without some effort or breaking them.

I was aware of people crowding around us. Someone was shouting for police. It might have been seconds, might have been minutes, I don't know because time stands still and flies all at once in such situations, but then there were sirens echoing and blue lights flashing and I knew the cavalry had arrived. Uniformed arms pulled at us, hauling us from our suspect. We were indignant. He was ours!

They didn't know we were plain-clothes cops and didn't believe us, initially.

Then the fire brigade turned up and an ambulance arrived, complete with stretcher. Turns out, the tube ticket man didn't know what I was saying or what I wanted so he'd called all three emergency services.

Our armed robber, Scott Benson, was nineteen and blasé. He'd robbed five bureau de change kiosks and had attempted to rob the one where we caught him. He came from a good middle-class family who were horrified.

At the station Benson said, 'I wasn't going to fire it. It wasn't a loaded gun. I wouldn't have shot anyone. I only wanted twenty grand then I was going to stop. This was the last one. Honest. I only wanted a quick buck.'

Because Benson had committed offences covering a number of policing areas, he would normally be taken down to the station where he was arrested to investigate and deal with it all. But a squad from Holborn had been collating the information on him, so they came to collect Benson and had the autonomy to deal with all the offences.

The DI in charge, far from being full of praise, told us off. 'What did you think you were doing, tackling him like that, knowing he would have a gun? You should have called for an armed unit. Idiots!'

'It was quick. We were there, on the scene, at the time. And we didn't have a radio, sir,' said Barry.

'Why the hell not? What do you think you're doing, going out without a radio?'

'There weren't any, sir,' I said. 'And not having a radio is no excuse for not doing our job. With respect. Sir.'

'So you played Dempsey and Makepeace, did you? Well don't bloody do it again.' And we were dismissed.

At least our own DI was impressed. And we didn't have to buy a drink for a week.

I read in the *London Standard* that Benson pleaded guilty and was given ten years in prison. The judge commended all the officers involved for their tenacity. Then he said this: '*I commend the two officers who apprehended the armed gunman for their bravery.*'

Barry and I have yet to see our commendations. I'm sure they loiter somewhere in the archives of a certain DI who was once in charge of a robbery squad.

B for bingo

There had been a series of burglaries in a block of offices in St James, so we had to make a plan. It was the same team in action each time, no doubt about it. The MO was entry through the fire exit.

Money was missing from desks, the coffee tin, the birthday fund, a sponsor money envelope and various other office collections. Milk from the staff fridges was finished off and the empty cartons left on the work surface. Biscuits and store-cupboard snacks were eaten. But the worst things about it were the deposits left on the desk of the company boss. Quite revolting. It was rather a gruesome find for the poor man. I'm sure these days DNA could be obtained but in the early 1990s it wasn't possible to extract DNA from faeces. The scenes of crime team scoured the offices for fingerprints but found only smudge marks, indicating the burglars wore gloves.

There were twelve offices in the block and each weekend for the last five weeks they had been burgled. We collated evidence and intelligence – method of entry, property stolen and so on. Armed with the information we arranged our operation. It was going to be a long weekend, starting 6 p.m. Friday through to 6 a.m. the following morning, then until 6 p.m. Saturday and the same Sunday. We would do this for as many weekends as it took. We had three teams of two – one pair in a car outside, one pair in the target building, and the third pair in the opposite offices with binoculars who were also tasked with keeping the log.

When you spend long hours on observations with someone, it helps if you get along otherwise it's not so good. The conversation can become as stale as the air. Once the 'what you did today' and the 'what you're going to do tomorrow' chat is over, there's not a lot to talk about so you end up talking about your families, your relationships, your lifestyle and your past. It's easy to see how some officers develop close friendships. Plus, any food brought along is usually eaten early on in the shift, often for the sake of something to do. And sorry, but really, I have to tell those partners who lovingly make sandwiches – they are regularly forgotten in favour of a fast food snack! If it makes you feel better, however – you can guarantee that halfway through chomping on a mouthful of pizza or burger or rotten kebab will be the time you get the eyeball and have to *go, go, go,* spilling hot coffee or fizzy pop down your shirt along with fried onions, greasy cheese and no end of other detritus. It's no wonder cops suffer with indigestion. Years of shift working and on-the-job scoffing fast food while on the run is no healthy diet.

Barry and I had the observation car on the Friday night. We used his private vehicle as mine was otherwise off the road; the ringer situation was still not yet sorted and no way would I use it for obs.

I smelled Barry's tuna sandwiches as soon as I sat in the passenger seat. This was going to be a long night.

We watched the last people leave and lock up the front doors of the office block at half past six. Gary and Matt radioed to say they were going up to the top floor of the building. Jas and Max were in the offices opposite and told us they had a great view of the fire escape and they'd just tucked into a Chinese takeaway.

By 3 a.m. the streets were deserted and there were no people left to watch. We were bored. At 6 a.m. we went home, nothing to report.

On Saturday night Barry and I were in the opposite building, binoculars and event log at the ready. We noticed the fire escape door on the top floor was open. Max and Jas were adamant it had been closed that morning when they left. Perhaps the cleaners hadn't properly closed it? Maybe the wind had blown it open? Bit far-fetched but plausible, at a stretch.

By midnight, boredom had kicked in. Barry and I were sitting comfortably in our obs point, waiting for the kettle to boil. At least we were warm and had a toilet for those necessary breaks. Barry cracked open the pack of digestives and we started a game of I spy.

We picked stupid things like CG – coffee granules, PC – paper circles from the hole punch, RIC – red ink cartridge, DITWD – dress in the window display, and ROTEOTP– rubber on the end of the pencil. Such obscure things kept the brain working even if we knew it was unlikely the other person would ever guess the objet d'art.

I was looking through the binoculars onto the street below when I had a eureka moment. I shot up straight. 'I've got it! I've got it!'

'That's clever, I haven't even said the initials yet,' said Barry.

'C!' I said.

'See what? What's happening? Give us the binoculars.'

'Nothing's happening. I mean C, that's the initial. Can't you guess? Dunno why we didn't think of it before.'

'It's not your turn. You didn't get *apple pip*. Err . . . I spy with my little eye something beginning with BF.'

'No. Not I spy. Can't you guess? It's bloody obvious!'

'What? Give us the binoculars, woman!'

He jostled me to grab them.

'Here,' I said, handing them across. 'But you won't see anything. Apart from Max having a fag at the top of the fire exit.'

Barry took the binoculars and watched as Max stamped out his cigarette and went back inside the building.

'Hasn't it clicked yet, Barry?'

'I'm not guessing. It's my turn, BF.'

'The burglars. No prints, just smudges. Nothing but money taken, easy to slip into a pocket. And the fire exit. Easy to leave it slightly ajar to make it look like that's how they get in. I guess the suspect is something beginning with C . . .'

Barry turned to look at me.

I saw it register in his expression.

'Ash, I think you've got something. But weren't they checked out?'

'I don't know. Think they were dismissed because of the timings. But it's easy to make something look like it isn't. I bet one of those offices have been done when the staff come in on Monday morning.'

Sure enough, one of the companies reported money left out by the staff had disappeared, along with a box of chocolates that had been eaten. Instead of a deposit on the boss's desk, this time it was in the waste bin beneath his desk.

Rather than six of us spending another weekend on obs, we convinced the DI to let us put in a hidden camera.

B for Bingo.

We caught our man. Sure enough, he was one of the C for Cleaners.

A couple of months earlier, Customs and Immigration had rounded up the cleaners on the office block. Two of the men were illegal aliens working under aliases. They were arrested pending deportation back to Somalia. A teenage cousin had taken one of the vacant jobs. He took the food for the hell of it, he took the money because he could, but the deposit was malicious, a deliberate defecation.

It was the boss who had tipped off Immigration and the motive was revenge.

Game on

We received information that a black saloon car was hanging around one of the parks near a school and the driver was picking up young girls. We needed to do some observations.

It was a cold Friday afternoon when I watched the black car pull into the parking bays near the swings. My stomach fluttered like a thousand birds. He was back.

I knew he couldn't see me hidden among the pile of stinking wood and rubble that had been there for ever, but I was nervous and anxious all the same. The stench of rotting materials seeped into my clothes and up my nose, along with the awful stink of damp old dog. I knew I'd smell like a tramp by the time I finally had a hot shower and washed it all away, off my body and out of my hair, everywhere but out of my head because it's never out of my head – it's always there, flashing unbidden like cards being dealt fast, the images of the people who do these things, the faces of the men, the women, and harshest of all, the screwed-up pained faces of the children.

He stepped out of the car and reached into the trunk for a ball, black and white, in support of Newcastle, or Notts County, or Dunfermline. He could be from anywhere like that because for all we knew, he wasn't from around here.

They never are.

He bounce-bounced the football around the park, playing keepy-uppy. One kick, two kicks, three. He dribbled the ball, keeping it tight in his control. I snapped the first photograph of the day to add to the collection from earlier in the week.

Any minute now she'd appear, bunking off school, tie loose around her neck like the long hair that flies free behind her. A pretty girl, a little chunky with pre-teen puppy fat, a trouser leg with a loose hem that flapped against her non-regulation cheap supermarket trainers. She's late. He looks at his watch. Kicks the ball against the back wheel of his car. And again. Harder. I feel his anger, palpable, like the bubbles inside my stomach.

And there she is. I take another photograph, this time of her. She's taken to wearing a little make-up: mascara and pink lip-gloss. Such a pretty girl, if only she believed it herself. They never do. Hers is a familiar story. She thinks she's fat. Useless. A chump with few friends. Any friends she did have were left at primary school and these kids she goes to school with now don't understand her and life's not fun anymore. Then she meets him, the guy in the play park, one afternoon when she bunks off, sick of the taunts and worse. He sees her and thinks she'll do. He talks to her, makes her feel good about herself and tells her she has such pretty eyes. His eyes twinkle at her so she believes him. This guy offers her something she's never had.

If this isn't her story, it's something like it, because it's one of many variations on a theme. A girl ripe for the picking, someone vulnerable, and these guys can spot kids like this with ease.

She approaches the car. He opens the back door and leans inside. He brings out two pashminas, one pink and one white, both with tassels and silver strands that glint in the dull sunlight. Gifts. Again. On Tuesday he gave her a couple of CDs. The day before that it was a magazine and a bar of chocolate that she slipped into her pocket.

She drops her bag by the back wheel, the one he'd been pummelling with the ball. She smiles at him and he bends to kiss her on the cheek.

I take another photograph. Catch him as he catches her, on the lips. Today would be the day. I know it. She's swapped the down-at-hem trousers for a skirt, black and pleated and hitched up higher than school allows. He strokes the back of her bare thigh and I click the camera again. I've seen it all before. Different guys, different girls, same story.

He takes a length of her dark blonde hair and she smiles at him as he curls it around his fingers. He bops her on the nose with the end of the strands and she falls into his chest with her head tilted to one side. She puts her arms around him, a shy bear hug. I see the sneer on his face and I know he knows he's won. He needs no more proof and neither do I.

It will be difficult to convince a jury because they don't know how it works, the grooming, and he'll give a credible story as he weeps in the dock. More reason to make sure the case is tight with little room for manoeuvre.

He pulls away and I see her look up at him with a fleeting look of fear like she's done something wrong. But he smiles and she relaxes. He opens the front passenger door and she slides into it. He leans in to click her seatbelt into place and I photograph it all. He kisses her on the lips, his hand lightly brushing hers. She has delight written across her face because she doesn't yet realise.

As the car departs, I reach for my radio. I flick the button on the side to knock it off mute. I whisper even though I know he can't hear me.

I repeat the message louder. 'It's game on.'

We have a duty of care, to protect, to prevent crime. We can't watch him groom her and then allow him to take her away. We know what he's up to, though of course, he will deny it. That's when our hard police work really starts: proving it.

The other team catch him. They stop his car and she starts to cry. He starts to swear, to object, he's done nothing wrong. He was arrested on suspicion of being about to commit a serious crime.

I video interviewed her but she said nothing apart from how she loves him and he hasn't touched her and she doesn't want him to get into trouble. It's classic grooming. I tried to explain to her mother, and to her, what a dangerous predator this man is but grooming wasn't an offence back in the 1990s.

Our suspect was a sex offender with convictions for assaults on young girls aged eight to fourteen. There was a lot on the intelligence log about him. He worked away from his local area, travelling from Kent. He was one to watch, to keep under surveillance, but with limited budgets and few resources, I knew it was unlikely to happen. It's not as if the operation would result in a drugs haul or bring some other major crime result. Police forces are always strapped for cash, and sex offenders are rarely high priority.

We did a little of bit of crime prevention that day; he didn't get to abuse that girl, and his cards were marked, again. But there was no 'result' that the bosses liked. There was no conviction because we had no willing victim that would go to court. We all knew what he was up to and knew he would continue to pick up young girls. Thankfully, the law has changed and there are Sex Offender Orders and many more offences have been created to cover crimes like this. He will have come to notice again without doubt. And if he's still in circulation and not in prison, at least he'll be monitored.

The beano

A team of armed robbers we had under surveillance decided to take a jolly. Three of them were in court on drugs charges and the other opted to stay in bed. As our day had gone awry we decided to go on a beano of our own.

Door knockers are rife in coastal towns and affluent suburbs where the pickings are rich and the antiques older than the oldest resident. Door knockers pick on the elderly, the confused and the wealthy, but just because these people might be able to afford such luxury items, it doesn't mean they should be fleeced. Many didn't even realise they owned possessions of such worth.

Door knockers have charm and patter and smooth dapper clothing to match. With their slicked-back hairstyles, fat rolls of money, and easy chit-chat, they impressed the old dears and conned their way into the homes of the vulnerable and confused. They picked their targets well and would do a recce of the property with a bit of their own seedy surveillance. They would work alone, or sometimes in teams, and would share information between them. If one had a good hit and there was more to be had, they would pass on the information for a cut. It could get quite territorial and turf wars were not uncommon.

They operated simply enough by knocking on a door and

charming their way into a house, then giving it the once over for anything of value. With their keen eyes for sharp detail, they knew what they were looking for. When they found it, they'd offer a paltry sum.

For something worth £500 or more it would be a case of, 'I'll take it off your hands, love. Fifty quid? More than it's worth really but I'll be doing you a favour, getting it out of your way.'

For something worth a grand it might be, 'Hmm, not sure it's worth much but I tell you what, throw in that vase and I'll give you a ton. It's a bargain. I'm doing you a favour, love. It's coming up for Christmas so just think what you can buy the grandkids.'

Conmen extraordinaire, they would take the booty to the auction houses of London and sell it to the highest bidder.

Our job was to gather intelligence and build up a dossier for the squad who would deal with them. Professional door knockers are anti-surveillance, savvy and sharp, because like all apprentices, they learned their craft from their masters.

In the absence of an armed-robbery team, we followed the knockers down to the coast. It wasn't easy. On this day they travelled in two cars. As soon as they hit the motorway, they doubled back on themselves, just to see who was following. They'd shoot off at the last minute at a junction, and would eyeball cars as they passed, clocking their registration numbers. We had a team of three cars and took it in turns to hang back, to overtake and ignore them as we drove by.

We hung about while they went to various addresses. When they met up in a pub we had ice-cream and then chips, as we waited. They'd had slim pickings that day and left empty-handed but we could place them together and had some addresses to add to the log.

Perhaps they planned to go back another day, to work on the victims some more, as they weren't biting. They had a habit of slagging off their colleagues and telling the unsuspecting pensioners the other bloke they'd had round was trying to fleece them, that the goods were worth twice as much as he'd said. It was all an elaborate con.

On the way back to London, the knockers called into a café on the roadside. Our team followed while I filled up with petrol.

One of the suspects clocked our third car as they pulled into the car park. He said something to his pal and they didn't stop; they were off, without waiting for their bacon butties.

It didn't matter. We had what we needed for that day. If they had clocked us, it might put them off for a while. Their lulls never lasted too long. They can't help themselves. They always come again.

For me it felt like a wasted day, a boring day, but some days were like that. Nothing much happened at all. We ended up collating information for future evidence, case-file compiling, and it was tedious work, but I suppose not every day can be full of excitement. We'd burn out even quicker. Though we did get a day beside the seaside even if it was more 99 than 999. With a flake.

Busted

Jaymie Tyndall had been under our surveillance for more than a month. We'd followed him, taken photos, knew who his associates were, which vehicles he used and where his lock-up was.

We had officers ready to pay a visit to his address at 6 a.m. one cold Monday morning. We knew he was in there because we'd seen him go in at 11 p.m. the previous night and the obs team watching hadn't seen him come out.

We hammered on the front door, armed with a warrant, the door buster and officers situated at the back of the house.

No answer.

Just as we were about to put the door in, a call went up from the rear. Someone had run out of the back, half naked, no socks or shoes, into the garden and straight into the arms of the waiting PCs.

It wasn't Jaymie Tyndall but it was someone we'd been on the look-out for. Good catch!

Rather than costing the taxpayer any more money by putting the door in, we entered via the open back door. Jaymie's mother stood in the kitchen, a thin dressing gown pulled around her scrawny body. Jaymie's sister, Darcy, came down the stairs, hysterical and shouting at us to get out of their house. She wore a velour tracksuit, her hair high upon her head in a pineapple ponytail, half a dozen gold hoop earrings dangling from her ears, and her fists covered in homemade blue ink tattoos. She looked the typical hard-knock gang member she was.

I told Mrs Tyndall why we were in her house and the rest of the team began the search.

'He's not here!' Darcy spat into my face.

'We think he is,' I told her, feeling disgusted at being spat it. It really is one of the worst things.

'Well think again!' she bawled.

Her mother lit up two cigarettes and handed one to Darcy. 'Calm down, our Darcy. They'll see. He's not 'ere.'

Darcy stared at me, defiant.

As they smoked their cigarettes, I caught a glance pass between them. I knew what that look meant.

I went to the upstairs. Darcy pushed past me and ran up them, two at a time. She stood at the top of the landing, hands on her hips, glaring at me. 'I tell ya. He's not 'ere!'

I shouted to the officers upstairs. 'Check the loft space.'

A female officer walked behind Darcy on the landing. Darcy spun round, grabbed the officer's hat and flung it at me as I made my way up the staircase. The hard top of the hat hit me on the temple and I stumbled.

Darcy flew at me and we fell in a bundle at the bottom of the stairs. I heard something crack and for a moment I wasn't sure whether it was her or me.

For once, it wasn't me. As we fell, Darcy's leg had twisted beneath her and broken. I felt a bit sick. It was horrible. Of course, she blamed me, and I certainly didn't feel good about it, but she'd flung herself at me. I wasn't sure what I could have done to stop it from happening. It wasn't good all round.

We found Jaymie Tyndall hiding in a space in the eaves of the attic. The wall had been boarded up to make it look like a natural plasterboard wall but it was really a hiding hole, complete with sleeping bag, torch and porn mags.

'Aww, man! How'd you know I was here?' he grumbled as he climbed into his clothing. 'Archie was supposed to lead you off. You got him then?'

'If he was your fall guy, yes,' I said. 'We got him.' We'd now got our man and another one thrown in for free. Bonus!

'Did he grass me?'

'No, he didn't. Let's just say I'm a dab hand at sign language.' I gave Jaymie the thumbs up.

You become quite familiar with the little signals and subliminal messages that people pass between them when you work with the public. This was long before the American drama *Lie to Me*, with Tim Roth, that great TV programme about psychologists who analyse body language to identify the secrets people, especially suspects, unknowingly give away, bounced onto our screens, but it's true. You can read people when you know what to look for.

Jaymie Tyndall plea-bargained at court and was given three years in prison for a variety of offences.

And it wasn't the last I saw of Darcy Tyndall.

Hats off

One of the saddest things I've ever had to do is to take a baby from its mother. It's always been necessary and it's always difficult.

Darcy Tyndall fell into drugs. It was inevitable as the people she associated with were drug dealers and users, her brother one of the worst. Her boyfriend was ten years older than her and well connected to guns, drugs and crime. By the time Darcy was sixteen she was a fully-fledged junkie with a hefty habit, paid for by petty crime and sexual favours to the drug-dealing friends of her married boyfriend.

Darcy was pregnant at seventeen. Her boyfriend dumped her. Her brother was in prison. All the agency professionals involved in her life hoped that she'd give up drugs. She didn't. She went through a spell of promising she had but when she gave birth, the baby was born addicted.

Darcy had a hard time in labour. Three hours after her son was born, the nurses found her shooting-up in the toilets, bleeding profusely and totally spaced out. The baby was incubated and safe. A strategy meeting was held at the hospital with police, social services, health professionals and others to work out a protection plan for baby CeeJay.

The following day, Darcy showered, dressed and picked up her baby for the first time. She bathed him, kissed him and told him she was going to give him a different life. She injected heroin then packed her bags. The nurses tried to stop her from leaving. She ran off with the baby to the toilets on the ward. I arrived with social services. She refused to hand the baby to the nurse.

I tried to appeal to her. 'He needs medicine, Darcy. He needs to stay here, for now.'

She didn't remember me. Not then. 'You're not having my baby! My baby!' she screeched, pulling him into her chest.

'If you don't let the nurse have him, I'll have to take him off you by force. Don't let's do that, Darcy. Please.'

She wasn't having any of it. After half an hour of pleading, CeeJay started to cry. One of the worst sounds is the keening of a drug-addicted baby. It sticks in your head for ever.

I had to wrestle the tiny five-pound baby out of his mother's arms as the nurses and a doctor and a social worker stood by watching. Only I could seize the baby under the Children Act, 1989, and place him in police protection to pass him onto social services, who would then place him in foster care until a court could decide the next appropriate action, all of which had to happen within seventy-two hours, maximum.

Darcy went onto have two more children. Her mother was granted custody of them all. And Jaymie's son, when Jaymie was found dead by the side of the road one morning. He was thirty-one. No definitive cause was found. He may have overdosed, or his body may have given up, or he could have just died. His girlfriend had been killed five years earlier in a car crash along with other drug addicts, and their poor children had only a grandmother and Darcy, their aunt.

However, I am really very happy to say that today, fifteen or more years later, Darcy has turned her life around. She is an ambassador against drugs. She's smart and intelligent, like she always was, and she teaches kids about the horrors of drug addiction, what it did to her and her family, and what it could do to them.

It had taken until she'd reached rock bottom and was on the streets for her to do it. I don't know what exactly the final point was but I knew she'd overdosed and nearly died; well, she had died but had been resuscitated in hospital after taking a bad bout of heroin that had killed a dozen or so addicts over a few weeks. Shortly after that, while still in her mother's care, one of her children became seriously ill. Maybe it was a combination of the two things or something else altogether, but she did it.

I'm proud of her, though I'm not sure she would want me to be. I was part of the system and she hated the system and everyone in it. But hats off to her. I'm so pleased she's done it. She must have saved so many kids from a life like she had. It's hard when you can't save them all but I know she'll be there to help them pick up the pieces when they need her.

Ménage à trois

It was a warm and muggy Saturday night in May. Soho was filling up like a boil, hot and sweaty and about to burst. Theatres were packed. The pubs spilled out. The tube trains writhed underground like fat worms. Leeds had been playing and fans were commiserating or celebrating, all loud and drunk.

It was my first shift of a week as night-duty detective. DC Sean O'Kane gave me the first job.

'Glad you're here, Ash. That armed robber is back. A tom's been done in Rupert Street. Can you go and see what she has to say? Looks like he had an accomplice this time. Let's see if we can nab these guys,' he said.

There had been a number of robberies involving prostitutes and allegations of rape by a suspect who was black, six foot and who wielded a good left hook as he held them at gunpoint. Everyone was on alert and everyone wanted him caught. It filled the working girls with fear. The girls took beatings by punters and were sometimes fleeced by guys who took themselves a freebie, but this was different.

I read the initial report on the CAD message. Two males had entered the basement flat of a prostitute and threatened her with a gun before being chased off. Young and white.

White?

Not our guy then.

I arrived at the address as DC O'Kane radioed me to say a taxi driver had phoned in. He'd seen two lads running down towards Shaftesbury Avenue being chased by a bouncer. The lads had legged it onto a number 25 bus and he was following behind in his taxi. Follow that cab!

I went to the flat and entered a tiny lobby. The stair carpet was worn, grubby, and more than a little sticky. At the bottom of the stairs a door opened to the left, into a reception living room, complete with sofa, portable TV, bookcase, table and fridge. No window. The fuggy stale air had a hint of knock-off perfume and it made me gag. I saw Francine De'Graaf sitting at a small round table adorned with a lacy tablecloth. Her hands shook as she dragged on a cigarette.

'I was sure it was him. That guy. I panicked, sorry.' Tears welled up in her bloodshot eyes. She dragged deeper on her cigarette. The overflowing ashtray hadn't been emptied for days. Or maybe she'd been chain-smoking.

The minder, Mary 'Ma' Baker, a butch middle-aged woman sporting a flat-top crop, sat next to Francine, stroking her hand. Ma had a fat Alsatian by her side and it was lapping from a saucer filled with digestive biscuits melted in tea. 'Ma' the Madam kept a check on a few of the working girls and was someone useful for them to have around, especially with the dog.

Ma pulled out a chair and waved for me to sit down. 'Don't worry, love, Archie doesn't have any teeth. He won't hurt ya. An' he can't bark either so don't be scared.'

It was a reminder that the power of suggestion is often enough.

The reception room led into the bedroom, which contained a single bed, a large mirror set in grotesque gilt, and a set of drawers.

Off the bedroom was a tiny kitchen and a minuscule bathroom with a shower that, should it ever be used, you'd have to stand in the toilet bowl in order to get wet.

Francine nervously flicked the top of her lighter, click, click, click, as she pulled her flimsy wrap tight into her petite frame. Her make-up was smudged and she was far from the twenty-six years of age she advertised herself as.

'I really thought it was him you know, The Beast. He did Trace last week and she's still in a right state. But these were young. And white. Can't be him, can it? Sorry. I panicked.' She became tearful again.

'Don't worry. You've had a shock. You're upset,' I said. I gripped her hand and squeezed. I could sense the fear she felt. It was in the air, along with the fag smoke.

Ma made a pot of tea. I don't like tea but didn't feel I should argue. She splayed four digestives onto a plate and the dog gave them the glad eye as I prepared to take statements.

Francine ground out her cigarette and lit another. She started her story. 'It was just after eight when this lad came in. He asked how much. I told him a ton. He looked young, like it might be his first time, so I asked how old he was. He said ,"old enough". I don't like them young but I figure if they're old enough to have the balls to come in here, then they're old enough.' She looked at me, defiant. 'I won't touch them if they're under sixteen.'

'And then what happened?' I asked, taking notes, getting the picture.

'He tried to get me down, bartered a bit. I could tell he was nervous, hadn't done it before. He was sweating, nervy, not confident like.'

I could imagine.

'We settled on sixty quid and he said he'd have to come back 'cos he needed to go to the cash machine. I didn't expect to see

him again. Then dead on nine when Dan, one of my regular
punters, was about to leave, the lad come back. Dan was settling
up with Ma and this kid just walked in, brazen like. I was changing
me stockings and I told him he'd have to wait. He said he had
the sixty quid. I laughed. I could see he was mad at me for
laughing at him. Then he said . . .' – Francine took a deep drag
– '"How much for twosie-up?" I laughed again and another lad
walked in. He must have been waiting on the stairs or somat.
This one said a hundred quid for the two of 'em. I said something
like, "Look sonny, go home, I don't do kids and I don't do
twosies."'

She started to cry. She stubbed out her cigarette making
the other dead-ends spill onto the table and down to the floor.
She lit up a fresh one.

'Then . . . then he pulled a gun. This thing that he pointed at
me. And all I could think of was that guy raping the girls. Robbing
'em. And here was two of 'em. With a gun. I screamed. I know I
panicked. Then I heard Dan shouting. He must have scared 'em
off because next thing, they're running up the stairs and Dan's
chasing them. It sounds daft now. But, but it was that gun.'

Ma put the kettle on again and I slipped Archie a digestive
before realising he couldn't crunch it.

Francine blew smoke up in circles. 'Will it take long, love? Only,
tonight's a good night. Always is on Cup Final night. With coppers
sniffing about, you're losing me business.'

What could I say? 'I'll be quick as I can but a statement might
take a couple of hours. Might be after two o'clock by the time
we're done. Sorry.'

'No disrespect, love, but they can *smell* a copper round here.
This could cost me a grand. Or more.'

I nearly choked on my tea.

By the time I'd started Francine's statement, Ma had turned

away half a dozen punters. One guy was persistent. I heard raised voices from the staircase.

'You'll have to have a word with him, Frankie,' Ma said. 'He won't listen to me.'

Francine went to speak to her caller. When she returned, she said, 'I told him to come back in an hour. He's a regular Saturday night John. He's French and not used to being told no. Thinks he can pop in whenever he wants.'

Wide-eyed, I continued taking her statement.

Sean called me on the radio but the reception was fuzzy so he called Francine's landline. He told me they'd arrested two lads who matched the description of our suspects. Both were fifteen, so their parents had been called and he was waiting for them to arrive at the station. He asked me to get a description of the gun and ring him back.

'It was black. And shiny. And big,' said Francine. 'Frightening. I don't know anything about guns. It was a handgun type. Maybe a snub-nosed thing? A bit like what Clint Eastwood has in that film.' She didn't know which film.

All I knew was the gun wasn't a rifle, a shotgun or a machine gun.

When I told Sean, he said, 'We've got the gun. It's a bloody spud gun! I'll send someone down with it once we've bagged it. Get her to have a look, see if she identifies it.'

She did. It was the gun. It was enough to stop her shaking and chain-smoking. She started to see the funny side. She couldn't stop laughing when I told her the boys came from affluent families and lived in the rich suburbs of London. They'd told their parents they were staying at each other's houses but they'd really gone camping in a field. They'd planned on shooting rabbits armed with the spud gun. In the unplanned way of teenagers with lust on the brain, they decided it was about time to venture into the world of sex and rock and roll. They necked a bottle of cider for courage and took a trip to Soho.

It put a different perspective on things. What we first thought was a vicious attempted robbery-rape turned out to be two teenagers chancing their manhood with a prostitute, asking for a threesome and holding her up with a spud gun when she laughed at them. It didn't detract from the fear they'd made her feel though, and we still had to deal with it as a firearms incident because they'd made it an imitation firearm the minute they'd pointed it at her.

I finished Francine's statement and made a start on Ma's when the creepy Frenchman appeared again. Francine said she'd tell him to go. She took him into her room and in a matter of minutes, enough time for me to write the first paragraph of Ma's statement, she returned.

'Is he going to come back?' I asked, head down, still writing.

'No,' she said, as she rolled a bundle of notes into a tin on the bookcase. 'It's pouring down and he's been waiting a long time. When I told him you were still here he said he'd settle for a hand-job. So I finished him off.'

I gulped. Talk about a quickie. It made me feel a bit queasy and slightly soiled. I hoped she'd washed her hands. I finished Ma's statement in a hurry. Now Francine was free she was eager to get back to business.

It was just after three o'clock when Ma signed her statement and as she wrote her signature for the last time we heard a thousand bovver boots hammering down the stairs. The door burst open to a heaving crowd of Leeds supporters, complete with blue and white scarves. They filled the tiny flat. A roar echoed around the room as they banged on the walls and chanted something unintelligible. They wanted action.

The ringleader stood nine foot tall. So it seemed. He had fists like footballs and sported a shiny wet bald head.

He bellowed, 'I'm first.'

Ma stood up, all five foot four of her, and barrel-chested. I admit I cowered by the bookcase.

A voice from the back yelled, 'You go first, Andy, we'll watch.'

Someone else shouted, 'Threesy-up!'

I cried inside. *Nooooo!*

The boom of their collective approval thumped in my head. Despite earlier thinking I might be in the wrong job money-wise, I certainly wasn't thinking of a change of careers. I picked up my radio and called for urgent assistance.

The radio didn't transmit.

I tried again. And again.

Something must have got through but Sean couldn't hear what I was saying. My heart pounded in my chest. How the hell was I going to get out of this?

I reached for the phone just as it rang. It was Sean.

'Did you call for urgent assistance?' his voice came to the rescue, like we were in a James Bond movie.

'Yes,' I squeaked.

'The kids haven't come back have they? We've just bailed them.'

'No, they haven't. Could you ... err ... send some uniform down to come and get me? Please?'

'What's all that noise? Ash? Are you all right? You okay?'

The flat was bursting with blue and white football supporters that put me in mind of a bunch of drunken Smurfs, though I'd never seen drunken Smurfs. They were refusing to take no for an answer. One was helping himself to a drink from the fridge, one lay sprawled and snoring on Francine's bed, another was taking a pee in the toilet with the door open. We three ladies danced around like imps, swatting sweaty hands as we dodged out of the way.

'Just send the troops. Quick.' I think I may have said something about randy drunken Smurfs.

We were duly rescued to a burst of applause from the Smurfs who simmered down once the cavalry arrived. None of them fancied sobering up in a cell. I was just glad to be escorted out of the flat and driven away in the back of a panda.

The cost of an arrest

Somebody in some department somewhere in a police building on the third or fourth floor will have calculated the full amount of how much it costs when someone is arrested. I have no idea what that figure might be but I know it won't be cheap.

Each case is individual, unique and time consuming. Forgetting the cost of the investigation, concentrating on the arrest alone, the figure probably runs into thousands of pounds.

I arrest Jom Said for shoplifting. It's eight o'clock in the evening. Mr Said is from Somalia and he doesn't speak very good English. We need an interpreter before we can give him his rights and start to process him. The only interpreter who can attend the police station is Mr Khalid and he lives an hour and a half away. He tells me he'll be there for ten o'clock.

Mr Khalid arrives and we find out Mr Said is sixteen. He's a juvenile and that means we need an appropriate adult to be present when we interview him. Jom Said lives with an uncle who works night shifts. His uncle can't attend the police station so we have to call social services who say they will send an appropriate adult but it may take some time because they are short staffed and their emergency duty social workers are all at other police stations. They also have a family of five children to take into care so we either have to wait, or find someone else who might be able to do it. We phone the local vicar who sometimes comes to act as an appropriate adult but he's unavailable tonight. A youth worker we have used in other cases is on holiday. I contact social services again and we're put on the waiting list.

Jom Said requests a solicitor. We call the duty solicitor but he's busy. He has a quick chat on the telephone with his client and the interpreter. The solicitor, Mr Ahmed, asks us to call him back when we have an appropriate adult and are ready for interview.

When Mr Khalid informs our prisoner of the delay, Jom Said has a panic attack. Or it could be an asthma attack. He thinks he's having a heart attack but he isn't. We are confident he's panicking so we call the police doctor rather than an ambulance. The doctor is busy but will attend when she can. It might be an hour or more and she advises us to call an ambulance if Mr Said's condition worsens. Jom is placed in a cell for juveniles, which is slightly different from other cells though not that much; it's still a detention cell. He's placed on constant watch.

The doctor arrives within the hour and examines him with the interpreter present. She tells us the reason Jom Said had a panic attack. It is because he's worried we'll find out that he and his uncle are here in London illegally. He's frightened to go back to stay with his uncle because he fears he'll be beaten by him.

The sergeant tells me to contact Immigration. I leave a message on their answer machine.

A social worker arrives after midnight. He talks to Jom Said through the interpreter. It's late. Jom is tired and emotional. We phone Mr Ahmed, the solicitor, who talks to Jom again. It's agreed it's too late to do an interview now. Social services aren't happy for Jom to return to his home address but they have nowhere to place him overnight so it's decided by all involved that it's best for him to stay in custody. We agree to convene again in the morning. Jom needs the obligatory eight hours' rest anyway. Social services say they have to pass the case to the local office so it might be ten o'clock before we can expect anyone.

Mr Khalid has to attend court the following morning so he can't come back to the station. We have to find someone else to do the interpreting. It's too late to ring someone at this time so I'll have to arrange that in the morning when I come back on duty.

The duty solicitor is working all night so he'll have to pass the case on to someone else in the morning, too. He arranges for us to ring his office when we are ready and they will send someone down to the station.

The underground trains have finished for the night and because I was on a 9 a.m. shift I didn't drive to work, I took the tube. A night-duty officer has to take me to the end of the tube line where I left my car. Then I'll be able to drive the twenty minutes home. Because the night-duty PC has to transport me, it means an officer is off the busy streets for at least an hour and a half.

I crawl into bed at three thirty and set my alarm for seven o'clock. I should be on a late shift but I'll have to go back in for another nine o'clock start to deal with Jom Said. As my department are short staffed, I know I'll have to stay on duty until 10 p.m., unless I have another prisoner, or some other thing to deal with, which will mean I'll have to stay longer again. I fall asleep, dreaming of a weekend off in three weeks' time. I'm so tired that I dream I am sleeping. I am that tired.

By midday the next day we are ready to interview Jom Said. We have an interpreter, a social worker and a duty solicitor. I need another officer to interview with me. I find a willing probationer loitering on the stairs on his way to his refreshment break. He wants to go into CID so he's keen to help and he agrees to miss his meal break.

The interview room is small and stuffy with six of us in it. Jom cries. He cries a lot. He told us he stole a sandwich from Boots because he was so hungry. His uncle doesn't feed him so he has to steal food.

Everyone feels uncomfortable.

I explain the situation to the sergeant. It's agreed Jom will be given a caution for theft. Then Immigration contact us. They want to come and interview Jom. I complete the police caution and I leave the social worker, interpreter and solicitor to wait for someone from Immigration to turn up. Jom has another panic attack.

I write up my case file.

My sergeant is eager for me to get back out onto the streets. Theft reports are piling up and someone has come into the station to make a complaint of assault, if I could deal with that first, thank you. It's a GBH and needs someone who can take a statement for such a serious assault and CID day duty have all gone home. I'm the only one left who can, or will, do it. I've worked so many hours of duty in the last forty-eight that I can't count them off the top of my head.

I summarise Jom Said's case as best I can. Cost of the item stolen: £2.20. And then some.

The day I met Jennifer

I was working a very busy late shift. It was raining rods, the air more than damp. The day was dark and it was generally a day for cheesed-offishness. We'd spent hours running all over Soho and Mayfair picking up pieces of various lives that played out over the capital.

It started with a warrant. A squat doorman dealer shifted his feet across the sticky carpet of the brothel we'd just raided after a tip-off from a disgruntled punter. A hefty stash of cocaine was attributed to the doorman, unless he came up with a plausible story otherwise. The West End bouncer, suited up like a Kray brother, stood watching us with a small steady yellow flame poised over an unlit cigar. I could almost hear him working out the lost percentages in his head – his cut, the madam's, the tom's, and that of his boss.

'You gonna be long?' he growled, puffing on his cigar.

'As long as it takes,' I shot back. I didn't want to stay there any longer than I had to, smelling his sour underarm guff disguised with aftershave and the stench of sordid sex and fake Cuban cigars.

Half an hour later we conveyed the cocaine, the prisoner and a few hundred quid to the station. Our prisoner's solicitor phoned to say he was held up so it would be a while before we could do an interview. It would be just enough time for the police doctor to come and give Mr Coke-head something to calm him down.

The sad, sorry day brought out the bizarre and peculiar. A probationer had arrested a kleptomaniac student who was doing a thesis on classical composers. The guy came from rich stock and had no need to steal. Nonetheless, he couldn't resist as he loitered in the basement store of Tower Records. He slipped an almanac of rare musicians into his floor-length overcoat.

As I had a couple of hours to wait around for my prisoner to be ready, I agreed to assist in executing a house search in the suburbs of Hampstead. I liked to be helpful and I confess, I was nosy, and liked looking into other people's lives. It's a good quality for policing.

We returned from the thief's house with a van full of stolen books worth thousands of pounds. I left the probationer to log and record it all and went to take solace in a coffee.

The canteen was shut. My friendly uniform colleagues had supplies, and at risk of being told to sod off, I practised my best smile and checked my pockets for ready cash should they charge me.

I flung my paperwork down onto a table almost knocking over a redundant polystyrene cup, edged with teeth marks and housing dregs of cold coffee. Doodled-on scraps of paper littered the table, so I swept them up into a pile, in case someone should need them.

In the corner of the canteen, I noticed PC Ritchie, a burly ex-dog handler, head down taking a statement from a pregnant lady who was rubbing her bulging belly. I really hoped she wasn't going to go into labour. Not here. Not now.

It was no surprise there were motor accidents galore on a sour day like this. Not being a traffic sort of police person and preferring to deal with crime, I tried to keep out of the way of smashed-up cars and broken-down motors, but I could offer some assistance here.

'Would you like tea, coffee?' I asked them.

'Yes, please,' she said.

I looked at her belly and like a mantra I repeated, '*Please don't go into labour, please don't go into labour, please don't go into labour.*' I didn't want to have to deliver babies. We hadn't covered it at Hendon or in Detective Training School and I wasn't feeling particularly knowledgeable about anything maternity, though I had passed my first aid course and held a St John Ambulance Brigade certificate. I waited for the kettle to boil and hoped I wouldn't need towels. I watched her as she leant back into the plastic chair to ease her back.

'Are you all right?' I asked, concerned.

'So what did he look like, the other driver?' asked PC Ritchie, oblivious.

'I'm okay,' she whispered, blowing out her cheeks. 'The driver? The one in the red Mercedes? Rather plump, an attractive girl, blonde hair, maybe thirty or so?'

I listened in, or rather couldn't help but hear, as I made tea. I added sugar, just in case.

She gave me a pained thank-you smile as I handed it over.

It was then I recognised her.

'Are you sure you're okay? Have you been checked by a doctor?' I was concerned. And a little star-struck, I have to confess.

'Doctor's on his way.' PC Ritchie looked up at me, frowning. He didn't appreciate being interrupted. Nor did he like that every few minutes another cop walked through the canteen for a gawp. News in a police station spreads faster than a shadow at sunset and everyone wanted to see for themselves who the celeb in the canteen was.

'Yeah, but he might be an hour or more. He's over in Whitechapel and I'm waiting for him to come and examine my prisoner. It's going to be nearer nine before he gets here. What about casualty?' I suggested.

'And wait around for five hours? No chance,' PC Ritchie tutted.

'It's okay. It's my third,' she said, smiling through her distress. 'I don't think this one's in any hurry. I've still got a few weeks to go.'

Despite it being her third, I could see the look in her eyes. It said 'pain'.

'I'll have tea if you're making,' PC Ritchie interrupted, closing down further communication.

'Sugar?' I asked.

I made him tea and handed around half a pack of biscuits I'd found in the back of the locker. I had no doubt I'd later be accused of stealing them.

Forty minutes later the police doctor arrived. My prisoner was declared unfit for interview as he was climbing the cell walls. He'd be okay in the morning after a night courtesy of Her Majesty's Police Service.

I gathered my papers and signed-off duty. It had been a strange day – dealers, druggies, rich thieves and celebrity car crashes.

That was the day I made Jennifer Saunders tea, with added sugar, just in case.

Exciting boredom

Witness protection is the sort of close protection given to people considered to be at risk of being got at, intimidated or otherwise influenced, or otherwise nobbled, as it is known to us. At risk of being nobbled, got at. It's serious stuff. Sometimes these people disappear, never to be heard of again, unless the nobblers are reckless or stupid.

Temporary witness protection is sometimes used for witnesses or jury members, or perhaps a judge, in serious Crown Court cases and it ceases once the case is over. When there was a serious and real threat to the course of justice we had to protect anyone in the case who was involved.

For my first time doing witness protection, I was posted with a guy, Bruce, who usually worked undercover in south-east London. I'd never worked with him before. We made up one half of a team working together for as long as the trial lasted. If the case went on for more than a month, we'd be given a couple of days off, but otherwise we worked, slept, worked and slept, around the clock, looking after our member of the jury.

It was a complicated case of blackmail, fraud and kidnapping, and the trial was kept out of the press because in a previous trial the jury had been nobbled. There was a strong possibility of it happening again so a news blackout was ordered.

Our guy lived in south-west London, somewhere totally unfamiliar to me. He lived by himself in a modern semi in a quiet avenue. We had to protect him around the clock, and wherever he went, we went too, whether that was the supermarket for his shopping, the pub for a pint, the cinema, the library, anywhere and everywhere, with us keeping watch out of sight, ready to pounce should we have to.

One of the other jury members went off to Paris every weekend, a long-standing arrangement, and his protection officers had to go too, all four of them, on the job. I never got people like that to protect.

Our man took his jury duty very seriously and told us he wouldn't be going too far as he didn't want to cause any trouble or put anyone at risk. I wished he had ventured out, done something a bit exciting. He was quite boring.

I was lucky to be posted with Bruce. He had a small camper van, which was a lot more comfortable than my little Fiesta. I lived miles away from the location so Bruce arranged to pick me up from the tube station near to the subject's house. It also meant he got the mileage expenses whenever we had to go anywhere with our target, but I was happy with that. I wasn't so fussed on the driving anyway.

We got the unlucky shift, 7 p.m.–7 a.m., which meant we had to keep vigilant all night with no snoozing on the job because if anything was to happen, it could well be then.

By Thursday, our jury man felt sorry for us and said he was going to go to the cinema, for our benefit. We bought tickets for the film and sat behind him. Why he chose to go and see *Pacific Heights* under the circumstances, I don't know. It was such an intense psychological thriller. I was on edge for the rest of the night. It was a fairly uneventful three weeks, apart from the night when someone called the police to say there was a suspicious vehicle parked up with two people in it. Uniform patrol cruised by and asked us what we thought we were doing. Of course, we had to say the real reason and acknowledged we'd failed to remain incognito. We moved our vantage point thereafter.

The rest of the time was quiet, which is as it should be. The trial concluded earlier than expected and I was called at home to say this stint of witness protection was over. I never knew if the accused were found guilty because of the news blackout. I did, however, earn a lot of overtime. I was able to take two weeks off and book a last-minute holiday abroad, on my own. It was bliss, mostly . . .

Saving lives

By the time police are called a dead body has usually been dead awhile, long enough for it to be futile to attempt resuscitation. I'd been trained well when it came to dealing with death and I'm very pleased to say that sometimes, you *can* make a difference.

The first time I saved a life was on that holiday in Corfu, the two weeks away on my own I mentioned in the last chapter. It was peaceful but kind of scary being on holiday by myself, but I managed to relax and enjoyed the chance to switch off.

But then . . . two days before I was due to go home, I was in a bar, it was late, and I was debating whether to leave. Three young drunks lounged in the corner like lascivious lizards. One fell asleep and his mates left him there. When he woke, he staggered and fell. He banged his head on a table and was flat out cold on the floor. Blood seeped from the back of his head.

My first aid training kicked in. I asked the barman to call for an ambulance and I grabbed a handful of serviettes to try to stem the bleeding. I bent down and saw his pallor was deathly white. I couldn't tell whether he was breathing. I felt for a pulse and couldn't find one. I tried both wrists and his neck. I bent my ear to his mouth and there was nothing. His chest didn't move. I shoved the paper towels behind his head. No pulse and no breathing. I tried to ask the barman for help but he didn't understand.

'Ambulance. Hospital. Doctor. Please call for help!'

I think he finally understood when I pounded on the man's chest and blew into his mouth.

I don't know how long the ambulance took but by the time they arrived, the guy was breathing. He wasn't conscious but he had a pulse and his cheeks were a more natural colour. The paramedics strapped him into a trolley and carted him off.

I was shaking and felt a bit queasy. The barman poured me a drink but spoke little English so our conversation was stilted. I spotted a wallet on the floor. I picked it up. It contained a student ID card of the man who'd collapsed. He was three years younger than me and from Wales somewhere. I don't remember his name.

The barman shrugged his shoulders. He didn't want to take it. 'Hospital,' he said.

I didn't want to go to the hospital at two in the morning to see a stranger, even if I had just saved his life. He'd still be there the next day so I thought I'd wait until then to decide what to do.

I didn't sleep well and the following morning I was up early. I took a trip back to the bar, a good enough place to start. A holiday rep was drinking coffee and asking the staff questions about the night before. The man who collapsed was one of the guests at her hotel. I filled her in, as far as I could, and I gave her his wallet.

She thanked me and said I'd saved his life. He was in a serious but stable condition. His family were flying over to be with him. She didn't know why he'd collapsed but thought it might have been epilepsy. I debated going to the hospital, but for what purpose?

I left for home a day later, still a bit shocked and in need of company. It was strange to think the man might have died if I hadn't been there, the right place at the right time. Luck. Or chance. Head or tails. The spin of a coin. If I hadn't had all that experience of death and first aid and dealing with it, I could never have done it. Some things never leave you.

It came off in my hand, sarge

Yeah, yeah, you all know by now that I'm accident-prone. Like how I don't have to wait to be injured when I can do it myself. These days it's called dyspraxia. I've had the formal diagnosis, so it's okay, but back then, I was just known as incredibly clumsy.

One sunny September afternoon, Barry and I were searching a transit van parked up in Berkeley Square. We'd nicked the driver for van-dragging.

The suspect had piled boxes from the delivery van into the back of his van when the driver was in the restaurant trying to find the manager. Luckily, we were watching the action and able to nab the thief and rescue three dozen bottles of Veuve Clicquot.

We'd just finished conducting the search and restored the property to the rightful owner when I slammed shut the back door of the transit van. The whole pane of glass from the offside window fell out and smashed at my feet. Ooops! Another report to write for accidental damage.

It got to the stage that my sergeant, the grumpy one, was going to bar me from doing house searches because I always came back having broken something. But it wasn't always my fault! Some of the houses we had to go into were not clean, not tidy and not pleasant at all. If they didn't keep their houses decent, how was it my fault that things fell apart?

Like the kitchen drawer I opened and the bottom dropped out, scattering knives, forks, spoons and other assorted junk across the floor.

Or the cot I leant against that clattered down in pieces, which I then couldn't put back together again.

Or the television remote control I stood on and broke.

And the ladies' marital aid I moved out of the way when searching under a bed only for the bottom to fall off, spilling batteries that the family dog swallowed. Don't ask any further . . .

Then there was the marble cheeseboard I dropped on my foot, smashing both the marble and two of my toes.

The spectacles I picked up for one of our prisoners, of which one arm fell off and we had to tape it back on so he could read and sign the forms in the station a là Jack Duckworth.

The amount of lights I've flicked on that have popped.

Lifts I've been stuck in.

The hole punches I've picked up, scattering little paper dots everywhere.

The cups I've knocked over, half full or half empty, I was never sure.

Door handles. Filing cabinets. Staplers. Police radios. I picked up a dead cat in the street, once. I was left holding its leg.

Ergo, it was no surprise when at the Christmas dinner party, my place name was labelled: 'Ash "It came off in my hand, sarge" Cameron'.

Christmas confession

When I woke up I realised I was still drunk. However, I couldn't not go to work. I certainly couldn't not go to work on Christmas Eve. They would know I was hungover because they had been with me. Celebrating. And you can't not go to work because of a hangover. Ever.

To miss work due to alcohol was a no-no, a no-go, and it would mean Big Trouble. You had to work hard and play hard, especially in 'the job', what with it being macho and full of hairy burly men. Okay, they weren't all hairy. Most weren't that burly. But it *was* very macho.

Christmas Eve was a day everyone wanted off so to go sick when you were rostered to work was another reason to turn up, inebriated or not.

I took the bus to the tube station. I couldn't face the walk. It was eight stops on the tube to central London and then I had to walk to the police station. I could manage that. I hoped.

The boss had promised an easy day. We'd be finished by one o'clock. Maybe two. We didn't have to start until ten o'clock so I'd be all right. It would be all right. I tried hard to convince myself of that fact as I left home at eight thirty.

I managed on the bus but by the time the tube pulled into

Liverpool Street I had to rush off the train before the doors closed. Once it left the station, I threw up, on the tracks, not the platform. I tried to be considerate even when I was disgracing myself. Beads of sweat filled my brow. It wasn't a good look.

When the next tube arrived I walked onto it head held high and trying not to make eye contact with anybody who might have seen me vomiting.

I kept the bile down until I arrived at the police station. I rushed straight to the Ladies in the basement, near the locker room. As I hugged the toilet bowl, disgusting smells and stains prompted more heaving. It was a pleasure to be sick in private after the humiliation of the tube station. I washed my face and tried to disguise the waxy, yellowy skin by lathering on thick make-up.

I must have done a reasonable job of convincing the half-team that was on duty with me that I was okay. They never mentioned the stain on my Christmas jumper, or the watery eyes. Perhaps because they had watery eyes of their own. I wasn't proud of myself. It was a terrible state to turn up in but I wasn't the first, or the last. At least I had one up on Barry. He hadn't turned up and was on the missing list.

The sergeant sent us on errands to collect his Christmas gratuity gifts from various outlets in the West End and in return he let us go home just after one o'clock, his Christmas sack full.

I still had some things to buy for my own Christmas: the Chablis for dinner, the specialities for breakfast, and a few other bits. Jas suggested we take a trip to Oxford Street Marks & Spencer.

All was fine until we reached the food hall situated in the basement. Like sturdy soldiers, the glistening bottles of wine stood, standing to attention. It was too much for my fragile stomach. I heaved. I swallowed. My mouth watered in the way it does just before you are going to be sick. I coughed. Heaved some more. My mouth went dry, my stomach weakened.

I spied a trolley piled with empty cardboard boxes in the corner by the service lift. I knew I wouldn't make it up the escalator, through men's clothing, past the fancy Christmas gifts and out onto the street, so I ran to the trolley, making it just in time. Yellow bile poured and I was unable to stop my stomach catapulting its sour contents into the cardboard box that once contained six bottles of Chablis.

I heard Jas say, 'Morning sickness. She can't help it. Sorry. Sorry.' She continued to apologise on my behalf all the way out of the shop. I'll never forget the sympathetic faces of the shoppers and store assistants. How could I?

So today, to all those people in Marks & Spencer, and all those travelling on the Central line on 24 December 1994, I apologise. I am sorry for being so drunk and hungover and for throwing up very publicly. I apologise for being unprofessional in my duty and turning up for work drunk from the night before. I am also sorry for passing it off as pregnancy sickness, not least because when I was expecting my third baby, I vomited every day of the pregnancy. Just deserts, I guess some would say.

It is with a sorry heart that I beg forgiveness. Can you pardon a young girl this indiscretion that has been carried for many long years?

My superiority is sweetened. It was nothing on Barry. He'd taken a black cab home but had puked, then fallen asleep. The driver had to take him to a police station as he was unconscious, unable to be roused, and the police placed him in the detention cell especially used for drunks as Mr Anon. They may or may not have discovered his warrant card, but they kicked him out of the police station once he'd woken up, when he was very apologetic, as was the way back in 1994 . . . but that's his confession, not mine.

The call you're waiting for

I'd been away from the East End for six years when I got the call. It was a Sunday and I was on nights. I'd crawled into bed at eight that morning and had only just stirred at 6 p.m. when my house phone rang.

'Hello,' I said.

'You sound tired.'

'I am. I'm on nights. It's been a tough week,' I said.

'Have I woken you up? Sorry.'

'No. I was lying here trying to summon up the energy to get out of bed.'

'It's Kenny,' he said.

'I know.'

'How did you know?'

'I've been waiting. I knew you would call.'

'Really? How?'

'Dunno. Just thought you might. How did you get my number?'

'Ways and means,' he chuckled. 'What are you up to?'

'I need to get in the bath, have something to eat, then leave for work again at half eight. You know how it is.'

'I do. But I don't do nights now. I'm on a task force unit.'

'I know, you told me. At Christmas.'

'Did I? I don't remember. I was in a bad way at Christmas.'

I knew he was. I remembered. His wife had left him and he was lost. I'd bumped into him at a police Christmas party. I hadn't been sure I wanted to go as it was one of those many dos you get invited to every year; people move on and new people replace them and I didn't know who I would know. I'd suspected there could be a few faces I'd recognise, so when my friend Elisha said we should go, I'd checked my shifts. I was on a rare night off so we went.

I'd bumped into Kenny and we chatted for nearly two hours. It was good to catch up. When Elisha and I left, we dropped him off at his new bachelor flat. I was driving and it wasn't much out of our way.

After Kenny had left, Elisha sat grinning in the front passenger seat. 'He likes you,' she said.

'Give over. We're friends. Well, we used to be. He's a good cop and a nice man. I just hope he's okay.'

'Yeah. But that's not the last you've seen of him,' she'd said, with a smug look on her face. Elisha always was a bit of a match-maker. She was blissfully happy with her man and wanted everyone to be as content as she was.

'I've told you before. I don't want to go out with a policeman. I spend all day with them. I want an uncomplicated man.'

Famous last words.

I arranged to meet up with Kenny in a few days' time when I had some days off. I joked I worked incognito these days and was he sure he'd recognise me?

He said the sweetest thing. 'You've always been with me. I've never ever forgotten you.'

Aww! How lovely! I was touched deep inside my heart.

Then he said, 'Every time I look down and see the scar on my thigh I remember . . . that was the night I was with you and I got my one and only injury ever. When I was stabbed with a toasting fork.'

Ach. That's Ash Cameron for you. The Angel of Doom.

I met up with Kenny. That was twenty years ago. The rest is history.

Animal lovers

People sometimes do the most disgusting things. I don't know how emergency service workers stay sane. Or why they are continually surprised.

Many of us have heard the stories of the orange stuck up somebody's bottom. Or the hoover nozzle fixed onto a penis. Perhaps the frozen sausage that was stuck inside a vagina, a severe case of freezer burn?

I'm not sure anything prepares you for the stories I'm about to reveal. The majority of the population would be horrified if they knew the awful stuff we had to witness, including the cruelty to animals. The only way we coped was with gallows humour and then trying to block it all out. You wouldn't want those images in your head for very long. Please feel free to skip. Nobody will know. If you decide to read you will have to excuse the terminology and the names we gave these criminals – people like 'horse-shaggers'. It was our way of dealing with it all. And I truly don't mean any offence to you when I write about them. Perhaps some things are better not mentioned at all . . .

Stanley the Stallion

I would love to use the name given to this particular man but the term is somewhat offensive. However, it is was what he was commonly known as. His real name had a certain ring to it, if you pardon the bad-taste pun, but for the purposes of publication, I shall call him Stanley the Stallion.

Stanley was arrested because he was caught on video in a farmer's field as he was standing on a milk crate committing an act of terrible indecency.

The farmer had been suspicious that his horses were being interfered with, so he rigged up his own secret surveillance. He caught Stanley bang to rights.

When interviewed, Stanley's defence was, 'But it was a female horse.'

The magistrates didn't take that into account when they gave him community service. Many mocked and said he'd already done his bit for the local community. He was hounded out, ridiculed, until he skulked back to live with his parents a few years later.

He was thereafter known as Stanley the Stallion.

Dirty Don

One of the local perverts was Dirty Don. For years he lived in his little house on his own. He was distinctive with a shock of white hair and beetle-black eyebrows. He walked with a stick and carried an air of superiority about him. Folklore said he used to be a schoolteacher until he was sacked in the 70s for touching up sixth formers at the convent school.

We received an allegation that Dirty Don had been flashing in the park that was used as a through route for the kids at a nearby comprehensive. Apparently, he was sitting on a bench reading *Moby Dick*. His stick was by his side, a pair of gloves next to him, his trouser fly open. Exposed and curled up on his lap like a sleeping snake sat his penis.

I asked Sophie, one of the 14-year-old girls who had seen him, to describe the incident.

She said, 'We were walking through the park and he was sitting there on the bench. I often see him sitting reading.' She detailed his clothing and what he looked like. There was no doubt it was Dirty Don. Then she said, 'I'd never seen one before. It was cold. I thought he should cover himself up.'

Bless her.

I called round to see Don with my colleague, Dave, to find out what he had to say. Don didn't want to let us into his house but when I said I was sure he didn't want to discuss his business on the doorstep and that we might have to call our uniform colleagues, he relented. I told him that instead of coming with us in our nice unmarked police car he would have to go in a police van and I reminded him how inquisitive neighbours could be.

'You'd better come in then,' he said, grunting at us.

His house was sparse but clean and tidy. He walked into his kitchen. 'I won't be a minute. I'm putting my shopping away.'

I followed him to make sure he wasn't going to go straight out the back door. On the work surface stood a bottle of milk, a loaf of bread and ten packets of liver. Ten!

'Lot of liver, Don,' I said.

'I have cats,' was his curt reply.

'Even so . . .' I said, my mind whirring.

We interviewed Don at the station. He denied being in the park or 'exposing his person'.

Dave asked him how he was getting on with *Moby Dick*.

Don said, 'I haven't read it for years and years. It was a set book when I was teaching.'

When Dave told him he'd seen a copy on top of the magazine rack by the side of his armchair, with a bookmark at page 172, Don blushed. He knew we had him. He admitted to being in the park.

'My fly might have been open, perhaps, but if so, it was an accident. And I had nothing on display. You know what teenage girls are like. Over-active imaginations.'

Out of devilment, I'm sure, Dave asked him, 'So, Don, what's the empty can of air freshener for, the one on the floor by your armchair?'

'Look here! What I do in my own home, by myself, is up to me. Keep out of my business!'

He was quite right, of course. It was none of our business. I'd seen the aerosol can with the bottom carefully removed, the edges smoothed down. A perfect receptacle, once packed with liver. Hardly Eau de Lady Garden though.

Dirty Don was found guilty by the magistrates. He was given a six-week suspended sentence, a fine and banned from local parks. I wonder if he ever finished reading *Moby Dick*?

Importuning and all that

The seedier side of the West End is hidden among the bright lights of fancy hotels, the glitzy façades of huge department stores and wafts of pungent garlic from the best restaurants. However, should you go loitering in certain parks and public toilets, you're sure of a big surprise.

We frequently received complaints about suspicious male activity in parks and toilets and when there was a flurry of allegations and objections, it would be time to concentrate on tackling the problem proactively, much in the way we did prostitutes and kerb-crawlers. Soho had a healthy and vibrant homosexual community and please don't think I mean to disrespect any of that. The things we were called to deal with in public toilets were often difficult and sometimes it was hard to distinguish between those who were genuine guys and those who were out to abuse other men.

Word would quickly travel around the 'cottaging' community that the cops were on the job and the suspects would disappear for a while, but we only ever succeeded in moving the problem on. We'd never ever stop it. They would transfer to different locations – Hampstead Heath, Wimbledon Common, and the other usual places for importuning, cottaging and dogging, then gradually gravitate back.

Today, the Internet makes it easy for like-minded folk to hook up but before computers and mobile phones, people took chances, risks, the anticipation and the frisson of meeting a stranger adding to the excitement and the thrill.

Whenever we did undercover work in relation to male sex offences, I obviously couldn't be part of the main team, and I was grateful. I was part of the back-up team and that suited me fine. We'd keep obs from a distance. We'd watch men enter the toilets, making a note of how long they were in there, watch for anyone else going in, and when they didn't come out within a few minutes in went the boys. They'd usually be caught indulging in some sort of sexual activity. If anyone tried to leg it, my partner and I would be there, outside, waiting.

The majority were married businessmen, influential and professional men, and some celebrities. They had a choice – admit the offence and accept a caution, or not admit it and go to court. A caution was an easy way out – confidential, out of the media, and hidden because nobody but the police knew about it. If they went to court, it would be on public record, perhaps in the newspapers. Many didn't want that. Regulars were charged to court.

Too much information is not always a good thing. Whenever I read about someone making an allegation of robbery or assault while walking their dog across a notorious public common, I can't help but wonder if it was an approach that went wrong.

It's good that society views all of this as different today. It's not a disgrace or shameful to be gay. It's perfectly acceptable to be with whoever you wish. People don't have to skulk or be embarrassed about who and what they are and they don't have to go to seedy places to find love.

There will always be predators and people looking to abuse, and people looking to pay for sex, but they are in no way similar to those genuinely looking for a partner.

Daisy chaining

It was one o'clock on a chilly night duty when Barry and I heard a call about a disturbance near Hyde Park. We'd just driven the unmarked police car along Park Lane and it was quiet, but Hyde Park is vast, so where to start?

A year earlier a tourist had been raped in the bushes bordering the park. The area was also becoming a habitat for drug dealers, and with druggies came robberies and assaults. Neither was it unusual for night-time filming to be taking place by wannabe directors and crew.

Barry looked at me and I looked at him, and we knew what the most likely cause was. A little bit of jiggy-jiggy. I only hoped it was the consenting kind.

The park was shut, all gates closed. The public toilets were empty. We asked the CAD room for more information, not happy to leave it as 'area searched, no trace'.

A minute later another call came from an anonymous person reporting a man in distress near the Queen Elizabeth entrance.

Barry drove to the gates, headlights shining down Serpentine Road. We couldn't see anything but as I wound the window down I heard a groan from the bushes to the left. Barry swung the car around.

We caught a group of men in various states of dress. They paused, looking like startled rabbits in the headlights. They hurriedly climbed into jackets, stuffed shirts back into trousers, straightened up ties and flattened down hair.

I climbed out of the car, shouted, 'Police!' and flashed my warrant card. 'What's going on?' I needn't have asked. Daisy-chaining.

'Nothing, miss,' said a tall gentleman with tufty silver hair. He fastened the buttons on his long mohair coat. 'We've just come from dinner at our club. We are walking hame.'

He actually said 'hame'.

Barry scrabbled in the back of the car for the torch. He flashed it at the men. One of them looked familiar. I struggled to place him. Did I know him? Was he on the telly? Had I arrested him before?

An older chap, head down, his bald patch shining, stood in front of another man but not before I saw the one behind zipping up his trousers.

Mr Tufty assumed the role of spokesman. 'We fancied taking a shortcut through the park. But it's closed. We were deliberating what to do when Hugo needed to empty his bladder.'

A police patrol van pulled up, lights much brighter and bolder than ours, and I saw a pile of assorted briefcases behind the men, stacked neatly and deliberately out of the way. Evidence of their spoils lay pooling on the ground.

Barry shouted, 'You're all nicked! Gross indecency. Get in the back of the van.'

'I beg your pardon, young man!' protested the older balding chap. 'Listen here. We are minding our own business. Mind your own. We're on our way.'

'Doesn't work like that,' said Barry. He wagged a finger, counting the men. 'Six of you. In public. In full view!'

He threw them the caution and I'm so glad he did, though nothing intelligible came back in reply.

With the aid of the uniform officers we bundled the protesting men and their briefcases into the back of the van and took them to the nearest police station.

They fluctuated between silence and mad protestations. Interviewing them we felt a mixture of despair and frustration.

We interviewed Mr Tufty first.

'The fresh wet patch on the ground, between you and your friend, Mr Wilson?' I asked him.

'Don't be silly, officer. I know the difference between semen and urine,' he scoffed, exhaling stale whisky breath across the interview table in my direction.

'What makes you think I don't? And I never mentioned semen,' I said.

He blushed.

Two of the prisoners gave false names but we discovered their real identities when we searched through the files in their satchels. Perhaps it wasn't surprising that they would attempt to pervert the course of justice by giving rogue details, considering one was a Crown Court judge, another a barrister, and the one I recognised – the clerk of the court.

They were all of previous good character, it was dark with few people about, and although in public, they had made attempts to be out of sight. These things were all factors that allowed the inspector to give them all a formal caution and a warning not to be caught again in public.

I don't know if they or anyone else notified the bar, but the Crown Court circuit is huge. Our paths never crossed again.

A pounding

I was working with our new sergeant on the crime squad, a large jovial man of Jamaican descent called Decca Decker, short for Derek. He was good to work alongside. He was funny, warm and generous, and a great replacement for the sour-faced, sour-breathed grumpy sergeant who preceded him.

Decca's knowledge of policing procedure, as well as his local knowledge, made him a walking, talking intelligence unit all on his own.

We were moseying through Soho on a slow walk back to the station when a short black guy with a tufty Afro walking in front of us suddenly jumped off the pavement and into the road. A taxi cab almost ran him over. He jumped back onto the pavement in front of two women walking towards him. He said something I didn't hear. The women gave him a strange look and sidestepped him, continuing on down the street.

We watched as he went into a closed doorway, faced the door and started fiddling with something in his hands. We hung back to observe him. I had no idea what he was doing; he might have been plain mad, or playing mad, but he *was* exhibiting strange behaviour.

A male couple, hand in hand, walked past him. He called them back.

'Here, come here!' he shouted.

They turned and went to him.

He huddled them into the doorway and showed them something in his hands. I didn't hear what they said but they walked off, apparently uninterested in whatever they'd been shown.

Decca said, 'Let's just give him a pull. See what he's up to.'

We approached him and before we could say anything, he said, 'Come here, come here.'

'What?' asked Decca.

'Have a look,' he said. 'I can give you this. For a price.' He opened his hands up. They were empty.

I began to think he was not quite sane.

Decca told him we were police officers and would like to search him to see if he had anything on him he shouldn't have. He said we'd seen him approach strangers in the street and he was exhibiting suspicious behaviour. In accordance with GO WISE policy, as part of the stop and search procedure implemented by the MET, we gave him the Grounds for the search, the Object of the search, produced our Warrant cards and Identified ourselves by giving him our names and police numbers. Decca told him which Station we came from and explained the Entitlement to a copy of the search. He could apply for it from the station within a year of that day.

Decca tried to herd him towards the doorway so he could start the search.

The man refused to give his name. He wasn't having any of it.

'Oh no you don't! You can't stop me. You can't search me. I know my rights. I've done nothing wrong,' he said.

'It'll take a couple of minutes and if you don't have anything you shouldn't have, you can go on your way. Just mind the traffic,' Decca said.

'You think you're so funny, don't you, big man?'

Decca asked him to take his jacket off but he refused.

'Look. It's simple. We can do it here on the street, which won't take long, or you can come to the station and we'll do it there. Your choice,' Decca said, smiling, as pleasant as he always was.

I reached out to reassure the man, as he seemed very agitated. I rested my hand on his arm and he flung it away. He stepped forward and pushed me. I stumbled backwards and he pushed me again. I fell against a shop window, which rattled and clattered and I thought I might go through it. I didn't like the look of the window display. It was a kitchen supply shop, with knives, scissors and wooden chopping blocks presented neatly in the front window.

He pushed Decca and turned to me. He punched me in the upper arm. I gripped on to the windowsill to stop myself from falling backwards.

It took Decca less than a minute to restrain and cuff him and arrest him for obstructing police in the course of their duty and assaulting a police officer.

I have no idea why he resisted being searched other than he didn't want to be. He didn't have anything on him that he shouldn't have. His behaviour was certainly odd but he wouldn't have been arrested for that unless he was causing a nuisance. And I had a hefty bruise on my upper arm, but I'd had worse.

He finally gave his name as Benji Obuya. He was charged with obstruction and assault and sent to magistrates' court.

Obuya didn't turn up at court and the case was heard in his absence. He was found guilty, fined £100 and ordered to pay me fifty pounds compensation.

He appealed the conviction and we were listed to attend Knightsbridge Crown Court for the hearing. In the meantime our legal department found out that Obuya was a member of an anti-police group and he was suing us via private prosecution for stopping him and depriving him of his freedom. He had successfully won two cases against the Metropolitan Police in the previous three years.

Sergeant Decker and I knew our case was watertight and the judge commended us both on our knowledge of PACE (Police and Criminal Evidence Act 1984) legislation. The appeal was lost and the penalty increased. Obuya was ordered to pay costs; his fine was increased to £500 and compensation of £100 was to be paid to me.

Obuya pleaded poverty and was allowed to pay a pound a week.

I'm still waiting.

Cassie's girls

There were certain places where guys who wanted underage girls would go and madams or pimps would provide. We discovered Cassie pimping her daughters on the streets like beggar children, waifs in need of proper love and affection rather than being skewed by the immorality of their mother.

Cassie had put all her daughters on the pill when they were ten. She said it was the right thing to do. Why the local health authority allowed it I have to question. Maybe Cassie thought she was protecting her girls by ensuring they had contraception, should it be necessary. In her world, it was the right thing to do. Surely someone should have asked why?

Cassie was twelve when her own mother died. The day after that, her father started to sexually abuse her. He continued abusing her, as did her two brothers, until the day her father dropped dead of a heart attack when she was eighteen. She hated him, she said, and willed him to die. She thought it was her fault and she had made it happen. It was etched in her face whenever she spoke of him.

Cassie's first husband almost beat her to death. He was violent sexually and physically, and emotionally abusive too. He was the father of Cassie's eldest two girls. He only left them when he was sent to prison for life for the murder of woman he picked up hitchhiking.

Cassie's second husband was the father of her third daughter. Then she had a son. He fell from a window and died when he was a few months old. It was deemed to be a tragic accident. Cassie's second son died a cot death. Her husband left her and that's when she started working the streets.

I knew some of Cassie's history and cut her some slack. I felt sorry for her, hearing her tales of tragedy and woe. But then we caught her pimping her girls and I no longer felt sorry.

Cassie's daughters didn't realise what they were doing was wrong. Their mother had been brought up with no concept of sexual morality, so I suppose I shouldn't have been surprised when they said they were just earning a living, a decent wage by decent means. They didn't get it. They didn't understand. They didn't know life wasn't supposed to be like that.

Cassie lost her girls permanently. They ended up in foster care and Cassie ended up living on the streets. Another sad life, a sad existence, and a terrible tragedy of abuse spanning many years. It was like a blessing when she died. She finally had peace.

And now Cassie's girls have daughters of their own. I hope it isn't too late to change the legacy.

Courting

Police officers spend a varying proportion of their time in court. Every person that is charged with an offence is sent to court and if they plead not guilty there is a trial. Police officers have to give evidence of the offence, anything they may have witnessed, details of arrest and interview and any other thing deemed necessary.

It used to be considered good practice to attend court for every appearance when your cases were listed at Crown Court. You needed to be on hand for the barrister, the CPS, the judge and your witnesses. You might turn up for what you think is a guilty plea, only to find the defendant had changed their mind at the last minute so a new date has to be set for trial and the available dates for all your witnesses should be to hand. A plea-and-directions hearing might result in the defendant changing his mind and confessing his guilt, so the court may decide to proceed there and then. You need to be on hand to provide up-to-date antecedent information.

Some great detectives taught me, and one of the best pieces of advice they gave is that you must know your cases inside out. Every scrap of information could become relevant. Most of it won't but you don't know until a sharp barrister in court asks you for it. It's embarrassing and unprofessional if you can't give an answer and court time is wasted while you try to find out.

As the officer-in-the-case, you need to be aware of bail conditions and every aspect of the case. It's vital to be able to furnish a judge with correct information for somebody they are going to sentence. If you don't, a smart defence barrister will soon correct you.

These days, with cost cutting and changes in policy, officers only go to court for the bare minimum of time and as a result, they don't get the experience and knowledge and aren't as involved in the cases as officers used to be. I have no doubt cases are lost as a result. Call me old fashioned but I believe it shows professional integrity to see it through every stage, not least for the victims. Nobody knows the case like the investigating officer.

I've given evidence in lots of Crown Courts: Southwark, Snaresbrook, Middlesex, Knightsbridge, Inner London, Isleworth, Chelmsford, Luton, Winchester, many in the North, and of course, the Central Criminal Court, known as the Old Bailey. Then there are magistrates' courts aplenty, and juvenile court, family courts, civil courts, the appeal court and the Coroner's Court.

I grew to love court work as I developed professional relationships with lawyers and CPS personnel. They knew they could contact me at any time and I'd try my best to help. Barristers have called me while I've been on holiday abroad with my family and in hospital after an operation. I know many officers would never dream of being available like that, but I've never had a problem with it, in the interests of justice. It was never a nine-to-five Monday to Friday job to me and if it made the difference between a watertight case and someone getting off on a technicality, there was no question: of course I'd assist wherever I could.

I've received a number of commendations for the quality of my case files from judges in Crown Court, a testament to the high number of convictions secured.

If you leave a loophole, a worm will wriggle through it.

The verdict

Everyone wants to go to the Old Bailey, the most prestigious court in the land. I lay claim to two cases there.

The first time wasn't exciting at all. It was a disqualified driving case that was only there because of an overspill in another London Crown Court. I was primed and eager to take the stand in my best suit. He pleaded guilty. All that and no trial, no giving of evidence, no swearing the oath in the Central Criminal Court.

It's always good when a defendant pleads guilty but this was the Old Bailey. I wasn't sure I'd get the chance again.

I did. The second time was very different.

A European girl, Celia, had a place at one of the best dance schools in the UK. She'd been in London for three months when a sadistic monster picked her off the street and raped her. She delayed reporting it for two days because she was ashamed, shocked and distressed, a very understandable reaction, especially as she was alone in a foreign country.

We found the perpetrator through DNA. His name is etched in my brain. Aggio Carribo. He denied everything.

The trial was listed for five days at the Old Bailey. Celia flew over from her country and we put her up in a hotel. She was as strong as she could be. She gave evidence in open court because the application for screens was dismissed, successfully argued against by defence counsel.

I sat in the police assigned area and cried as Celia cried. After her two days in the witness box she flew home.

The following day the defendant stood in the dock, with a puffed-up chest like a proud peacock as he gave his evidence. He said Celia consented to have sex with him.

The jury found him not guilty.

What they didn't know was that he'd been to court twice before on rape charges and had been acquitted then, too. Same MO: young foreign girls, vulnerable and easy prey. Who knows how many others there might have been that he plucked off the streets and that weren't reported?

I had to ring Celia and tell her the jury failed to convict Carribo. It was a terrible phone call. All of that angst and distress and reliving her terrible experience in court for nothing. She vowed never to come back to London. I couldn't blame her.

Carribo was free and would probably do it again.

Contempt

We had a trial listed at Knightsbridge Crown Court that was due to start the Monday after my holiday abroad. It was a three-handed street robbery team that we'd had under surveillance for a few weeks. We had a lot of intelligence information to back up our operation and we caught them in the act. They were sent to court and pleaded not guilty.

Kenny, my partner, and I arrived at the airport to fly home in plenty of time. Our flight was due to leave late Saturday night but it was winter and there were fewer holidaymakers and so the airline had merged two flights. I hadn't checked the times as you are advised to do. Our flight had been cancelled and everyone had been transferred onto the earlier one. We were stranded.

This was years before budget airlines started up, and the flights to Spain left for England during winter on Saturdays, Tuesdays and Thursdays only. There was no guarantee we would both get to London, or even be on the same flight. It was a case of taking whatever we could get, whether it was Bristol, Manchester or Glasgow.

I contacted my office on the Monday morning for somebody to pass a message onto court. I was horrified when they came back and said the judge was mad as hell. He agreed to postpone the case until Wednesday, but if I wasn't back by then he'd hold me in contempt of court. Did I realise how much public money I was wasting?

I felt bad. Really bad. And panicky. What if we couldn't get a flight? We couldn't even get a hire car to drive back because neither of us had thought to take our driving licences.

I spent two anxious days flitting between wanting to get drunk and worrying about being banged up in a cell for a week, courtesy of Judge Waterhouse.

The relief when we managed to get a plane to Luton was immense. I didn't care that we were sitting at either end of the plane. I'd have gone in the hold if it meant getting home.

The robbery trial lasted a week and the defendants were all found guilty. The judge sentenced them to between three and five years each.

Afterwards, over a drink in a nearby hostelry to celebrate, our barrister told me I needn't have worried. The court list was packed on the Monday and the trial wouldn't have started until Wednesday anyway!

Through the square window

It's hard when you have child witnesses that have to go to court and give evidence. Today they don't have to do it in the courtroom because it's done via video link. The child sits in a specially designed interview room somewhere else within the court building. It's still very stressful for them to relive their experiences, especially during cross-examination. It's horrible. When a child is accused of lying, some cry. Juries are often told by defence counsel that they cry because they were lying and have been caught out. That's not true: they cry because they are distressed, upset and have been accused of lying.

Abusers usually pick children because they are vulnerable and easy to manipulate. It takes a lot to stand up to an adult, especially one who has done terrible things to you. The people who abuse kids know it's easier to pick on those who can't fight back.

In my experience, the more vulnerable the child, the more you can trust what they say, especially those with learning difficulties or the very young who have no concept of such matters. They don't have it in them to make up things like that.

The youngest child I interviewed was four years old. Emily was a bright little girl who described in detail how her mother's boyfriend put his Charlie in her hand and how he made it be sick. Unless a four-year-old has previous knowledge, or has an exceptionally vivid and adult imagination, they could never make that up.

The boyfriend denied it. The CPS said she was too young to be put before the court and that anyway she might have forgotten the incident by the time it came to trial. They said to put her through the ordeal of giving evidence would have a detrimental impact on her and that she was of an age where she would probably forget all about it. This meant we had no case against him.

Thankfully, social services held a perpetration hearing in the county court. It's a case brought in the civil court where the judge decides, on the balance of probability, if something happened. The criteria are lower than in criminal court and if there is a finding of guilt, there is no punishment or conviction but it certainly helps when it comes to social services making decisions in the best interests of children as they can use these cases as evidence.

This was a rare move and I wished they could do it more often when the CPS didn't proceed with a criminal trial.

Emily didn't have to give evidence at the perpetration hearing, but the judge watched the video of me interviewing her and I was asked questions about the way I interviewed her. On the balance of probabilities, the judge was able to pass a finding of guilt. As it wasn't a criminal court, no sentence could be imposed, but it was sufficient to prevent him from having contact with children. If he ever did, social services could take positive steps to protect them.

Emily's mother chose to stay with her boyfriend, which meant Emily and her siblings were removed from their mother's care. She married him and the children were all placed for adoption.

A few months later, he almost killed Emily's mother during a domestic incident when they were both drunk. He was charged to court but she refused to give evidence against him. I daresay they are still together, fighting, abusing and being drunk somewhere.

Let right be done

I've had some good results, as well as some rotten ones. The psychology of a jury fascinates me, how they work, how they are influenced, where their own life experience fits into their decision-making. Are some easily manipulated and are others not that interested? Who takes the lead and why? Are they influenced by prejudice? Does a tenacious barrister influence or repel them? How much credence do they give to children's evidence? Why won't they convict mothers who hurt their own children?

Now the restriction on police officers and ex-officers has been lifted, I'd love to do jury service but I think I'd probably be a harsh critic. I know too much about how the court system works and I'd be critical of the police and prosecution because I could see between the lines and I'd also be wary of the defence barristers because I know their tactics. A hard place to be, should I ever have the chance.

I've dealt with offenders who have been sentenced to ten, fifteen years or more, such as in shaken-baby cases, rapes, GBH, indecent assault and armed robbery. I've been involved in cases where life sentences have been handed down.

Most of the sex offenders I investigated received imprisonment.

Some sentences seem harsh, others lenient, but they are decisions for the judge who has sentencing guidelines to follow and his or her own rulings to make.

A finding of guilt has to be beyond reasonable doubt, the jury absolutely sure. I know not every person in the defendant's box is guilty, but I've believed in every case I've taken to court. It's not for me to judge anyone. I could only put a case together with the best possible evidence.

I have stood up for justice on both sides. It has to be right.

There's a saying: 'It is better that ten guilty persons escape than that one innocent suffer.'

That is true. And in my experience, the guilty are caught out eventually and usually end up back in court.

In stitches

Times were changing, as was force policy. In the late eighties, the Met had gone from being split into four areas of policing, roughly north-east, south-east, north-west, south-west, to being chopped into eight. It was confusing. All to do with budgets and command units and things that didn't really affect the ground workers too much. They also introduced something called 'tenure' in the early nineties, which was basically about people movement. Five years in any one post was the maximum, the decision makers declared. Their idea was based on the idea that familiarity leads to complacency, corruption, laziness, burn out and other not-so-good things. In reality, some people *were* ready to move on after five years for a variety of reasons. However, making it blanket policy meant a huge loss of experience and local knowledge as highly trained officers were moved onto somewhere and something new. It takes time to be fully trained in each police role and you build up contacts, networks, informants and trust. Just when you became an expert, they were now going to move you on and train up new people. Ergo, a force full of Jacks (of no trades) and no Masters (of any).

Tenure was one of those in-house political procedures that we could do little about. All you could do was hope you were over-looked or given an extension for some exceptional reason, and that the policy would change before it was your turn.

My days were numbered, so rather than be pushed or poked into a hole I didn't want to fit into, I started to look in Weekly Orders (a weekly publication full of force information, e.g. people joining, transferring, retiring, and also any internal positions vacant) for new positions.

I found one. It was plain-clothes and detective work, and closer to home. I applied, was interviewed and got the job.

I transferred to the new Vulnerable Persons Unit, investigating domestic violence, some child abuse, all homophobic and racial attacks, abuse of the elderly and vulnerable, missing persons, plus anything else that came our way that didn't fit neatly into any other box.

I knew I would miss my old team. I'd loved working in the West End. I would miss the busy and exciting buzz of that sort of work, but things change. This was a positive move and would give me more experience.

I moved in with my partner, Kenny, at the same time as I changed jobs. We were restoring, modernising and redecorating. The day before taking up my new post was a grainy Sunday. It was drizzly and January cold. We popped out for a lunchtime drink and were home an hour later.

Neither of us can recall what started the argument. It was a silly thing. Something like who didn't put the milk back in the fridge, or who forgot to feed the cat. As I stomped off up the uncarpeted stairs, I heard Kenny call me a name. A bad name. I stomped back down, furious. Kenny stepped into the kitchen and slammed the door, unaware I was standing behind him.

I saw it coming but could do nothing to stop myself falling head first through the glass door. Hundred-year-old bevelled glass half-an-inch thick smashed into a zillion shards as my head split open and blood spouted in an arc.

Kenny grabbed a tea towel and applied pressure as my hot rich blood covered his hands. I remember thinking *I hope that tea towel is clean.*

It wasn't a good start. There was no way I could report sick on my first day. Despite a thunderhead, I turned up for work as expected. Kenny came with me. We stood in the office of my new boss, Detective Inspector Bolan. He looked at us with sceptical eyes, like two naughty children caught in the act.

'Honestly, sir, it was an accident. We did have a row but it was a total accident. He shut the door behind him and didn't know I was there. I went through it, couldn't stop myself.' I knew how it sounded. I'd heard it all before, many times.

'Hmm,' the DI said. 'You do know these are the excuses women give in abusive relationships? Women you will have to deal with?'

I didn't say, *men, too.* It was best I kept my mouth shut. I nodded. 'Yes, sir. I do know, sir.'

Kenny gave it a try. 'It really is the truth, guv.' He laughed. 'I wouldn't dare hurt her on purpose. She's got a helluva right hook.'

The Guv looked at Kenny, raising his eyes further. He turned to me. 'How many stitches, Ashley?'

'Six, sir, they come out next week,' I said, knowing I'd got my Sunday name rather than 'Ash', and it wasn't good. I wished I could kick Kenny, make him shut up.

The DI looked down at his papers and waved us away with a simple flick of his hand.

That afternoon as I was familiarising myself with the station, he found me and gave me a little talk. If there was anything I wanted to tell him, he said, his door was always open; he was there to help, no need to suffer in silence.

How cringe-worthy. The talk. The one I would say many times

over the course of my career to those people who had been battered and or abused by those who are supposed to love them. I wasn't one of those people, honest.

A few weeks later it was Valentine's Day. Kenny was on a week-long residential course for work. I sent him a card, with a poem. I sellotaped the six stitches across the top.

I think my DI eventually came to believe I wasn't a battered spouse as he discovered during my two years in the unit just how exceptionally clumsy I am.

The day Diana died

When Kenny and I had two babies, we decided to move away from London. A northern force was accepting transferees. We applied and were accepted. I'd been a police officer for nearly twelve years, my husband for longer. We both had to start from scratch, prove ourselves all over again, like newbies. It was demeaning and I felt it discredited our achievements. It was also a massive waste of public money to train us for things we already knew, like first aid, driving courses, diversity and more. I'd worked hard to get into CID and had done my time on crime squads, undercover work, murder investigations, domestic violence, vulnerable people and racial incidents, the like of which involved things that were unseen in this section of the naive North. It was the bottom of the pile for us.

We had two babies, one a few months old. The bosses put us on opposite shifts, no doubt thinking they were doing us a favour. It was hard. When Kenny was on nights, I had to bring the kids to work at 5.45 a.m. and hand them over to him in the station so I could do an early shift. He then had to stay up until 8 a.m. to take them to nursery. It was the same when I was on nights. Our kids were regulars in the nick at odd times of the morning and the evening. It's what we had to do. With nursery provision to pay for, the finances wouldn't work whichever way we tried it, so we both ended up working full time. Career breaks were frowned upon and if I wanted to drop any hours because I was a working mother, well, did I want to be a police officer or not? It was how it was back then.

The day Diana died, 31 August 1997, I was on night duty. It was a Saturday night/Sunday morning. After the rush of drunks refusing to go home and the subsequent domestic call-outs once they had, things had quietened down. At 4 a.m. I returned to the station to complete a pile of paperwork. I walked into the CAD room, the control room hub, and *Adagio in G minor* by Albinoni was playing on the transistor radio. It has always been one of my favourite pieces of music. When the DJ told the early morning audience about the accident in Paris, I was shocked. Dodi and the Princess. He was dead and she was critically injured. The chauffeur was killed and they weren't sure about her bodyguard. I sat, shaken.

I can't say I knew Princess Diana any more than any of the general public, but I'd seen her on plenty of occasions during my days in the West End.

I knew the private bodyguards who guarded Diana when she was with Dodi. They worked for Mohamed Al-Fayed who had offices in Mayfair. His protection men were well known to us in CID and the squads. They had the best CCTV system of the time. The team, all ex-servicemen and ex-cops, worked often with us and were all high calibre and highly trained. It was an exclusive position, working for The Big Man. I'd often wondered if he had a place for a woman on the team but I doubted it.

I finished my paperwork and went home at the end of my shift. Kenny was on a day off but the babies were up, unforgiving in their childish ways. He was watching television instead of listening to the radio, like he usually did. We watched the tragedy unfolding in France. I remembered the security guys well. Any one of them could have been there that day. At midday I went to bed a bit grief-stricken, and like much of the nation, I knew British history had changed. And no, I don't believe the conspiracy stories. Not all of them.

Women's work

I was pregnant for the third time in less than four years. My idea was to get childbirth all over with at once, fewer interruptions to life and to my career. Maybe it was a good plan, maybe not, but I didn't want 'the job' to think I wasn't serious. They didn't like women going off pregnant, interrupting the flow of things, even if it was only for twelve weeks, the maximum maternity leave at the time. It was just how things were then. I chuckled to myself, wondering what they would think when I returned to work, bringing expressed breast milk with me to store in the fridge.

While pregnant you have to do non-confrontational duties so I was put into the Admin Support Unit, also known as the Criminal Justice Unit. It was where case files were prepared for court. I sometimes had to take statements, which meant going to someone's house. It wasn't always safe but we made the job work and I wasn't going to refuse. I happily did things that perhaps in hindsight might be considered risky today.

Roy, one of the blokes in the office, had less than a year to go before retiring. He was another old sweat who thought women should leave the job when they have babies and he would shout it out to anyone who would listen.

Roy complained about me to the boss, Arthur Johnson. Arthur

was a retired senior officer, which is why he got the position in charge of the unit as a civilian when he left the job. Even though Arthur was no longer an inspector, I still called him sir. Roy told him I was coming to work grumpy in the mornings and it was upsetting his daily routine. He accused me of kicking the bin when I came in.

'I have no idea what he's talking about, sir,' I said, affronted.

'The complaint is that you don't like being here. That you'd rather be at home.'

'What?' I looked at him in amazement. 'I don't think that. I like working in this office. It's good to know what's going on in the courts and who's currently active, it's a great job for someone like me.'

I thought back to one morning the previous week.

'I think I know what Roy's talking about, sir. I came in last week five minutes late because my son had a minor epileptic fit at the breakfast table. He's prone to them. Rather than call in sick to stay home and look after him, I took him and his sister to nursery and came to work. I had my handbag, and my briefcase, and because I was rushing I'd forgotten to leave the baby-change bag at nursery. I was laden down when I came into the office and pushed the door wide. Roy's bin is behind the door and it was knocked over. I didn't kick it. I had a bit of a moan saying how these early starts are a struggle with being pregnant and having two little 'uns and how I felt guilty for not staying at home to look after my little boy when he was poorly.' I looked Arthur in the eye. 'With respect, sir, that's all it was. And I stayed until half past four, when I should have left at four.'

'I see,' he said. 'Well try to be on time in future. I suppose that's the trouble with being a working mother.'

The civilian staff in the office, of which there were plenty, were allowed to work flexi-time, so they came in at all times and left at all times, as suited them.

'It is a bit difficult getting in for eight o'clock, especially with morning sickness and my husband doing shift work. Is there any way, sir, that I can do flexi-time? Or do a nine to five instead of eight till four?' A reasonable request, I thought, and it wasn't as if I wouldn't get my work done.

'Oh no. Absolutely not! I can't let you do that. If I made an exception for you I'd have to do it for everyone and I can't have that. I'd never be able to keep track of who's doing what.' He shook his head as if I'd just asked the impossible. I suppose for him, it was.

'But the civilian staff work flexi,' I said, flogging a pointless request.

'Yes, because they're civilians. You are a police officer.'

I didn't know what difference it made in that office and I don't know what I'd expected, really.

'I know you work hard, Ash. Just keep your head down and out of Roy's way.' I was dismissed.

Out of Roy's way? I walked back into the office and picked up Roy's bin. I moved it to the other side of his desk. 'Don't know why you didn't move it before, Roy. Everyone comes in and knocks your bin over. Is that so you get a warning and can hide your football cards?' I smiled at him. I had his measure. I did twice as much work as he did and I know he booked out an unmarked police car to go and see his fancy woman because I'd seen the car parked outside her house a few times when he was supposed to be elsewhere.

When my doctor suggested I went sick for the last three weeks of pregnancy, it didn't take me long to make my mind up. Thirty-seven weeks pregnant, with a three-year-old and a two-year-old, and I couldn't keep any food down. I was anaemic and dehydrated. Hmm. Not a hard decision to make.

My daughter was three and a half months old when I returned

to work. I'd added some annual leave at the end of the statutory twelve weeks. I had a position in Child Protection to go to and I never had to work with Roy again. No doubt he was pleased to see me doing what he considered 'women's work'.

Mommy dearest

When I was midway through my third pregnancy I'd taken a couple of days' leave as my daughter was starting afternoon school nursery. I was looking forward to a couple of days' rest and being away from the old grouch in the office, Roy.

My little girl and I were stood whiling away the minutes before the doors of the school opened when I heard the crack of splintering wood, followed by a smash. I turned to the houses opposite to see a youth climbing into a garage through a broken glass window. I thrust my daughter at another waiting mum with instructions to 'Call the police! Tell them I'm an off-duty police officer and someone's burgling the garage.'

I ran across the road and hollered at the youth to stay where he was. He picked something up from inside the garage, threw it and broke the rear window. He made a swift exit into the enclosed garden. He couldn't escape because I knew the gardens backed onto other gardens, with high walls dividing them. I entered the garden through the gate and yelled at him, 'The police are coming.'

'Fuck off!' he shouted back as he made his way to the bottom of the garden where the bouncing begonias beckoned.

'You can't get out,' I shouted.

'Watch me!'

I had no intention of watching him. 'I'm a police officer, stay where you are.'

He made a running jump at the wall.

I lurched forward and grabbed his dangling legs.

He kicked out at me.

I held on to his trousers and pulled him down, a tad relieved I was wearing dungarees.

He lunged again, still struggling to escape.

'I told you, I'm a police officer.' Oh, and something like, '*You're nicked*.' He leant forward and I pulled my head away, having learned to avoid head-butts. He bit me. Hard. He sank his teeth into my hand like an animal and drew blood.

'Oi!' I screamed, and let him go.

He struggled to stand up and when he did, he grabbed me by the straps of my dungarees and swung me around on the grass.

'I'm pregnant!' I screamed.

'Good,' he said, spitting in my face. He kicked me in the stomach.

It hurt. I did the only thing I could. I rugby tackled him and fell on top of him. All fourteen stone of me.

He looked young, about seventeen. I could tell he was high on account of his glassy, pinprick eyes, and pale sweating body. I'd guessed I might gain the advantage by sitting on him but it didn't stop him struggling, pulling out clumps of my long hair, spitting and trying to bite me some more. I held on. He was going nowhere.

Finally, the police arrived.

Was it worth it? To be assaulted while pregnant? To have hepatitis and AIDS tests, again? I was bitten, I was bruised and I was battered, all while carrying my baby.

Gareth Harrison was given nine months in a young offenders' institution and ordered to send me a letter of apology. I'm waiting. I did get a commendation, though, which the chief constable forgot to include in the annual award ceremonies. Three years later, when I queried why I'd never been given it, my chief superintendent said sorry and he gave me the framed commendation himself.

It sits on my lavatory wall as a reminder.

What do you call it?

To be an effective child protection detective you not only need to have good detective skills and abilities, you also need to have a special child protection qualification. This means you have to go on a specific child protection course. I attended two, one in the Met and one up North. That means I must have been quite superb, really, doesn't it? Ha. I don't know about that but I like to think I did a good job and I helped some people.

Child protection training is carried out in conjunction with social workers and it's called a 'joint-investigation course' because child protection cases are jointly conducted with a police officer and a social worker. Both vie to be the lead professional but each come to it with different outlooks. I don't mean disrespect to either profession when I say social workers tend to minimise and police tend to maximise, so it's good to see things from each other's perspective, to round off police sharp edges and sharpen up social workers' round ones.

When I worked in child protection teams we generally had a very good working relationship with our social service colleagues and those in the wider multi-agency professions. People tell me it's changed today and that's a shame. Perhaps putting the CPU (Child Protection Unit) personnel – police, nominated social workers, health and education professionals – all in one place, and calling it a multi-agency child protection unit, might help the working relationships to improve but I'm not a policy maker and why should anyone listen to me? Maybe one day someone will have the same idea and make it happen.

The courses are comprehensive and intense. They instruct you on how to Achieve Best Evidence in relation to video interviewing of victims and witnesses, and the training covers lots of other things too. The lessons can be harrowing so the trainers try to lighten it up a bit with some silly but relevant activities.

One 'brainstorm' session after lunch had us in groups of three or four. We had to make a list of all the words, medical and slang, that we could think of that people might use to describe their private parts. How many can you think of?

We had 147 different labels on our list, a few I didn't know, and a few forenames because some are used to label private parts, such as John Thomas, Charlie, Mary, etc.

Those names I vowed never to call any child I might have. And some of the descriptive words, well, you just had to laugh.

Yet despite the 147 on our list, in reality there are many others that children use when interviewed and some that I'd never heard of. You have to be open, receptive and non-judgemental, and even if shocked, not to show it.

This sort of work would be miles away from the rufty-tufty grappling on the streets and undercover kind of policing I was used to, but those skills weren't wasted. As you will see . . .

Double jeopardy

We had an allegation of child abuse from a young girl who said eighteen-year-old Tim Abbott had indecently assaulted her for a period of about six months. He was a youth loosely connected to her family and they used him to babysit for her. The only address we could find for him was one that his family had moved from a short time earlier. As is the way in a community that hears whispers of things they don't like, word filtered through to us that Tim Abbott was hiding out at his older brother's flat on a new housing association estate. His brother, Ben, was twenty, known to police for a few minor offences but not known to child protection. We had no photo ID for either of them.

Trevor, a detective in my office, took a trip with me. After the third knock on the grubby front door of a maisonette, a short, dishevelled-looking, tufty-haired young man answered, wearing nothing but boxer shorts. It was just past midday and around the time that those with nocturnal habits start to rise.

'Hello, mate,' said Trevor. 'I'm DC Donovan and this is DS Cameron. Are you Ben Abbott?'

'Er . . . naw. Mate.' He scratched his left ear. 'That's me brother. Wot ya wan' him for?'

'Can we come in a minute?' Trevor took a step inside the half-open door, which he took to be an invitation to come inside.

'What ya want our Ben for?' the young man said, stepping aside to allow us into the hall.

I took a deep breath, not wanting to inhale too deeply inside the flat. I followed Trevor, my hand on the radio in my jacket pocket.

'Who are you then, mate?' asked Trevor, who had everyone down as his mate, unless they became 'pal', which was when his colleagues knew that Trevor was not feeling very pally.

The youth shut the front door and stared at us. 'I'm 'is brother.'

'Which brother is that then, mate?' persisted Trevor.

''is only brother. Err . . . I'm Tim . . .'

'Aah, Tim! Fancy getting some clothes on then? And we'll have a chat.'

'Worrabout?' Tim suddenly came alive. 'Hey! You got a warrant?'

'Don't need a warrant, mate. We only came by on enquiries and you let us in. If you get some clobber on, we'll have that chat.' Trevor's hand moved to his rear trouser pocket, the one holding his Kwik-cuffs.

'Err . . . yeah . . .' said Tim, walking backwards. 'Gis a min.' He entered a door at the end of the hall.

A minute passed. Nothing. Then came banging from inside the room.

'Balderdash!' shouted Trevor. He didn't really, but he did utter a rude expletive meaning the same. 'Bet he's climbing out the sodding window.'

Trevor tried to open the door but it was locked. He shouldered the panel door. The flimsy slide-along lock popped its screws and the door flew open to reveal the bathroom. Opposite the door was the bath, lengthways along the wall and half full of water.

Above the bath was a shallow but very long window, the width of the wall.

There was our suspect, clad in only boxer shorts, half-hanging out of the window with his legs dangling over the bath. The window wouldn't open any further.

'Stop right there!' shouted Trevor, as he leant across to grab the youth.

I pulled the plug in the bath.

Trevor yanked a dangling leg, stepped back and knocked me to the side. The suspect gripped on to the bricks on the outside windowsill and flailed his legs. As he did so, he kicked Trevor in the face, his heel smacking into his mouth. I jumped up and grabbed a leg, any leg, and pulled. With a tremendous splash and a heck of a commotion, all three of us tumbled down and over into the draining bath.

Trevor grabbed the guy and spluttered, 'Tim Abbott, I'm arresting you for indecent assault on a young female', and before he could shout out a caution, another semi-naked young man appeared in the bathroom doorway.

'Wha's going on? Gerroff me brother!' He took a step towards us.

The suspect in the bath shouted out, 'I'm not Tim! He's Tim. He's the one ya want! I ain't done no assault on no one. I was only kidding I wasn't Ben 'cos I didn't know what youse wanted me for.'

I looked at Tim in the bath. I looked at Tim in the doorway. They certainly looked like brothers but I had no idea who was who.

Trevor struggled up out of the bath while I kept hold of Tim-in-the-bath. Tim-in-the-doorway picked up the toilet brush and brandished it at Trevor. Then he made a run for the front door shouting, 'I'm not Tim! I'm not. I'm Ben. He's Tim.'

'Oh no you don't!' hollered Trevor, taking out his CS spray.

'Drop the brush and move away from the door, pal, or I'll use this CS spray.'

I have no idea how it happened and can only blame extreme confusion.

Tim-in-the-hall lobbed the brush at Trevor who in turn aimed the CS canister straight ahead and shouted, 'Spray! Spray!', and promptly CS sprayed himself, a direct hit in the face. It shouldn't have been possible as the spray comes out of the hole at the top of the canister in the direction you aim it. How Trevor managed to CS himself, he has never been able to explain. Thankfully though, enough of the gas managed to incapacitate Tim-in-the-hallway and he lay on the floor gagging and begging for his mum.

Although my radio was, like me, a tad waterlogged, I managed to call up for assistance and we contained both Tims, the one on the floor coughing up all manner of snot, tears and phlegm; the one in the bath, who had stopped resisting, probably because he was frightened I was going to submerge his head under a running tap or try to gas him. Or something. Not that I would do such a thing.

Keystone Cops had nothing on us that day but at least we got our man. Two of them, in fact. The real Tim for indecent assault and the 'other' Tim for perverting the course of justice, which was down-graded to obstructing police in the course of their duty.

Which one was the real Tim? I can't recall now . . .

Not their fault

Victims of sexual abuse are very brave to come forward and report it. Historically, the police haven't always been sympathetic as an organisation, and individual attitudes along with old-fashioned ideas made it worse. It's abhorrent to blame the victim, to say they're asking for it, that it's their own fault, that they could have stopped it, or to accuse them of making it up, but for some people, it's easier to believe the victim is lying than to deal with a difficult case.

Years ago, victims might have been given a hard time and have been told they would have a harder time in court if they gave evidence. They would have had to prove they were strong enough to withstand cross-examination. It wasn't only police that compounded this but the whole justice system.

Attitudes are much better now but there's still a long way to go in helping and supporting victims, especially the vulnerable, like children.

I've dealt with hundreds of allegations of abuse and sexual assault and only a small minority were made up, or false.

Prostitutes would sometimes claim rape if a client didn't pay. Technically, it was a making-off-without-payment offence, but selling sex isn't a legal transaction. These cases were a nightmare to deal with and the women were often referred to civil remedies. Sometimes, though, a prostitute *was* raped and because of her occupation it was difficult to secure a conviction. It would be held against her in the courtroom by Rottweiler defence barristers and juries who were not sympathetic. Nobody deserves to be raped, whatever life choices they make.

You need to gather as much evidence as possible to build a case and it's not enough to have one person's word against another's. Medical evidence may verify a sexual act took place but it doesn't always prove a case, especially when it comes down to a matter of consent. If the starting point is one of disbelief then the victim has got no chance. Sometimes the evidence helps the defence, sometimes the prosecution, but when you're investigating you gather all the evidence and present it as one package. You often don't know what's relevant and what's not until the court case and if you don't present the best evidence, how can a jury be sure beyond all reasonable doubt?

It's traumatic when children make allegations of sexual abuse. Paediatricians with specialist training in sexual offences conduct the medical examinations. It's horrid to think of children as young as three or four years old being abused. The youngest I dealt with was an eleven-month-old baby. The medical evidence stood where verbal evidence couldn't, and the abuser was given a twenty-year jail sentence.

Polly was a nine-year-old girl who had been neglected by her family. They lived in appalling conditions. She was taken into care and placed to live with an uncle who molested her. When I video interviewed her, she gave clear disclosures of sexual abuse by her uncle and a friend of his. Her hymen was broken, which confirmed her allegations of rape. She had anal tags, which helped prove an offence of buggery. She had a severe case of threadworms and a ball of worms was found inside her vagina. She was self-harming and exhibiting signs of anorexia.

I arrested the uncle and his friend. Both denied the allegations.

A psychiatrist said Polly was too fragile to give evidence in court and it would be detrimental to her emotional wellbeing. The CPS said we couldn't charge either suspect without our victim and it was unfair to put her through such a traumatic ordeal. If only there had been another way we could have dealt with it.

Social services red flagged both men, which meant that if they came into contact with children, the system should kick in and the children could be protected from them. But the system is not infallible. I know these guys are paedophiles and sometimes there's not a thing I, or anyone else, can do about it.

Mum's gone to Iceland

Ashley and Tracey, Cagney and Lacey. Our colleagues thought they were being funny, ha ha. But you need to have some laughs when the days are doom and gloom.

I had to make some enquiries with social services about a family that had slipped out of notice, so Tracey, the social worker, and I paid a visit to 6 Montgomery Terrace.

I knocked a number of times before the door cracked open.

'Mum's gone to Iceland,' said Amelia Fleming, looking at me with eyes that flashed teenage defiance.

'When will she be back?' I asked, hoping she meant the shop, not the country.

'When she's done, s'pose.' Amelia leant against the doorframe, arms crossed.

'When did she go?'

'A bit.'

She wasn't giving anything away. A baby cried from inside the house.

I pushed the door ajar and put my foot into the lobby. 'Amelia,' I said. 'Let us in. Please.'

She moved away. 'You'd better come in then,' she scowled.

We entered the house and the struggle was evident. Three

children under the age of ten sat quietly on the grubby settee, stuffing spilling out where it was ripped. Little legs with dirty socks hung over the cushions. Sallow eyes followed us as we walked around the room and took in the scene. Rubbish lay scattered across every surface. The smell wasn't pleasant; it was stale, and dirt and heat emitted from a calor gas unit turned to max. A packet of custard creams, Asda's own brand, lay open between two of the children. Their breakfast. A baby's bottle lay dripping diluted orange juice onto the grimy carpet. Cartoons played out on the small television, volume set to loud. It was a Wednesday; the children should have been at school, the youngest at nursery.

The baby cried again. Amelia left the sitting room and came back with her sister, eight-month-old Billy-Jo, a tea towel wrapped around her lower half as a makeshift nappy. A stained white vest hung open at the poppers.

'Mum went to get some nappies,' Amelia said.

'When did she go?' asked Tracey.

I saw the young girl glance at the hallway. Those subliminal signs tell a lot.

'Let's go upstairs, let the kids watch TV,' I said.

'No! You can't go up there. Stop,' shouted Amelia, moving across to the doorway.

I ignored her and took the stairs two at a time. The door to the bedroom at the front of the house had a tiny padlock on it.

Tracey and Amelia were behind me.

'Amelia, let us in that room please,' I asked her.

'No, I don't have to.'

She hugged the baby tight, tears coursing down her face.

I had a dreadful feeling, and a swirling in the pit of my stomach, familiar in these circumstances, started to gnaw at me.

'If you don't open the door, we'll have to put it in. We don't want the little ones to get scared, so please, why don't you open it?'

'No!'

I took her hand, held it firm and looked her straight in the eye. 'I know this is hard but I promise, we promise, we will do our best to help you. Please open the door.'

'You can't help,' she sobbed. 'You can't. It's too late.'

Amelia was thirteen. She had tried to keep her family together, bore the brunt when her mother couldn't cope. This time it was different. It would have been easy for me to push the door open but it was important that Amelia allowed us into her mother's bedroom.

Tracey held Billy-Jo as Amelia opened the lock. 'I had to put the lock onto stop the others coming in. I told them she was sleepin".

On the unmade double bed lay the body of Julie Fleming. An empty pill bottle on the table beside the bed had once held prescription tranquillisers for postnatal depression.

Amelia had done her best and my heart ached for her. They had been a family in need, a family who had been in and out of social services offices many times. Julie had been a child in the care system herself. They had been doing well but recently they'd been flagged up because there had been a number of failed appointments and the children had been absent from school all of the previous week. We knew there had to be a problem but it was too late to help Julie.

We had to find a permanent foster home for five children aged thirteen to eight months, hopefully together, as I promised. It was a hard job but we found someone out of town that would take all of them. Often they end up split between homes.

Mother love

The most precious thing is a mother. Allegedly. Having dealt with some atrocious mothers, I can't help but think how their offspring feel on Mother's Day. These women are very different from the women who struggle to cope or can't parent for whatever reason. Not everyone can. It's the malicious and deliberately criminal mothers that I struggle with the most. And as I've said elsewhere, it's often the kids who've been abused that love their abusive mothers and fathers the most. Some people don't deserve to be parents.

It's really difficult to convict a woman of abusing her children. For whatever reason, juries do not like to think about a mother inflicting pain or cruelty upon her own. It is even more difficult to convict a woman of sex offences. It's an uninhabited territory. There are many more women who abuse children than the general public realise. Even professionals have difficulty accepting it when the abuse is sexual. It is abhorrent to think about and for a jury made up of law-abiding citizens, it's beyond their ken. I understand that. It doesn't pay to think about such things, to allow your mind to wander to those dark places, so it's easier to believe it's made up, or that it doesn't happen.

I can't begin to describe the horror and the neglect Tracey and I faced when we turned up at a caravan site to look for a family of young girls nobody had seen for two weeks. I cannot list the all the concerns and everything we uncovered because if I wrote the summary of the case it would take a whole book, and it wouldn't make for comfortable reading.

The following chapter was my introduction to the family.

Fly away home

Five pairs of sad eyes looked up at me, sad faces with mouths closed and bodies defiant. They'd been taught to say nothing to social workers and police officers and teachers and they weren't going to say much today.

Our question, 'Where's mum?' was met with, 'Out.'

That's as much as we got. It looked as if mum had been 'out' for some time.

It was eleven o'clock in the morning. The one-bedroomed caravan was freezing. The girls huddled together by the front window, sitting on the tatty brown and orange cushions that made do for seats.

The littlest girl was three. She wore one of her older sisters T-shirts and a pair of rotten, once-white socks. Her big brown eyes stayed focused on me as she sucked on a dummy.

The eldest girl, Kim, was 14 but looked both younger and wiser than any 14-fourteen-year-old I've ever met. 'Mam'll be back soon. It's Tuesday, yeah? She gets her money today. She said she'll bring us some food.'

Two empty tins sat on the table, bean juice congealing around the rim, drips trickling down the side. The lids had been hacked off. An empty packet of cheap breakfast cereal was upturned; a few stale cereal hoops lay scattered.

'What have you had for breakfast?' asked Tracey.

'Cereal.' Kim pointed to the empty box.

I opened a cupboard and a door hung down off the hinge. There was a tin of tuna, a packet of tea bags, a bag of sugar spilling its contents and a tub of gravy granules. Nothing else.

'No fridge?' I asked, thinking the van itself was colder than most fridges.

Kim shook her head.

There was an open plastic milk container by the inset sink, an inch of sludge inside. I didn't want to get too close and I could smell it. I guessed the cereal for breakfast had been dry.

'When did you last have anything decent to eat? Like a proper meal?' I asked.

Kim shrugged.

Her lank dark brown hair fell down between her jaw and her collarbone. It looked like it hadn't been washed in a very long time, nor seen a brush. Then I saw them, saw something crawling in her matted hair. I focused on the top of her head, at the movement. Flies. Lots of them. Creeping and crawling about her head. She scratched just above her ear and I think she was unaware she was doing it.

I walked over to the other girls and looked down at them as they sat looking up at me. Two more dark heads and two dirty-blondes. They were all rife with head lice. I've never seen any so big that they looked like flies.

The girls sat and stared at Tracey and myself as we searched the caravan, looking for anything that could tell us where their mother might be.

The gas heater had no gas bottle and apart from a box of matches, there was no lighting once it was dark. The place was a tip and it stunk like the dirtiest training shoe. We couldn't possibly leave them in such a midden.

The caravan park, Dipden Hollow, was a known paedophile's paradise. When released from prison, or given bail from court, they moved to the caravans because it was cheap, easy and accessible. It was also full of DSS families who unfortunately were unable to secure rented housing. Picture-perfect for paedophiles.

We had travelled to the caravan park in Tracey's car, as she knew which plot we were looking for. There was no way we'd be able to fit the five of them in the back of the car. I was relieved, in a guilty, selfish way. I called for the police van to come and collect us to convey us to social services' offices

'Oh, and John, on your way up will you please bring five happy meals? I'll pay on delivery.'

Tracey told the girls, 'We're going to get you something to eat and find you somewhere nice and warm to stay until we find your mum. Why don't you get dressed. Who likes burgers?'

Kim, her eyes teetering with tears shook her head. 'We're not going anywhere. Bev told us to stay here. She'll be back soon.'

Bev. Their mother. To hear Kim talk of her as Bev told me so much. It would become more significant later, but even then, when she called her mother by her first name, I knew.

'Was she here last night?' I asked Kim.

She shook her head.

Bev hadn't been there for a few nights, was my guess.

The girls didn't have any clothes to put on. They had what they wore, which was very little. In the bedroom, on top of the stained double mattress, lay a jumble of clothing, dirty, damp and disgusting. I expected something to crawl out from the stinking bundle. The girls would have to come as they were.

What we didn't know at that time, and neither did they, was that Bev was in a caravan three plots down, wrapped up warm and cosy with a paedophile who was on bail, charged with rape and buggery of children under ten. Bev hadn't seen her daughters for nearly a week.

The girls were placed in foster care and gradually, when they were ready, they started to talk.

It was one of the worst cases I ever dealt with – neglect, physical and sexual assault – and with all of that came the inevitable emotional abuse. Bev couldn't see what she was doing was wrong. Or so she said. Despite all the girls making disclosures of their mother being present when they were abused, she denied it. The CPS said the case should be split into two: the eldest two and the youngest two – but the very youngest child was too young to give evidence. For me the case was more powerful with all of it together, every victim and every scrap of evidence put together with a myriad of offences charged. They said no. We failed to convict Bev of anything but she agreed to work with social services and undergo an in-depth assessment. She never got her girls back but now they are adults with children of their own. I saw them all together in town just the other week, Bev, with her grown-up kids and their kids. They saw me too. I could only walk on by.

Wearing his ring

Jemima had been violated. When we took her for the medical examination, the doctor confirmed her hymen was broken. We would surely have a court case. The perpetrator would be sent to prison, maybe, if he pleaded guilty, or was found guilty at trial. So many variables. What could I say to Jemima's mum?

'We can arrange counselling. If you feel she needs it,' I said.

'Oh yes. Sure. Bring it back to her for an hour each week and I'll watch her suffer the fallout. Until the next week. Same time, same place, and we do it all again. And in her head he'll be doing it to her all over again. Been there. Done that,' she said.

I'd heard this many times, and people have to want to talk for counselling to work. 'Maybe it'll help her. It does for some people.'

Mum slumped into her chair. 'Perhaps it'll be different. I should have saved her.'

'How's she coping?'

'She's petrified. Have a look on her left hand. The middle finger. That bloody silver ring with those stupid snakeheads. That's his ring. He told her if she ever took it off, she'd die. Doesn't matter what I tell her. She won't remove it. As soon as I saw it, saw her wearing it, I knew.'

I had seen it. Jemima told me about it when I interviewed her.

How do you convince an eight-year-old girl she won't die when it's in her head she will if she takes the ring off? It was beyond my abilities. She needed proper counselling. I knew before she told me that she felt dead inside, already, even with the ring on. It's a common thing to feel for those who've been abused.

'What do I tell her?' asked her mum. 'I was eighteen before I had the courage to take that bloody ring off my finger. Instead of throwing it away, I threw it at him. It's my fault. I didn't think he'd do it to her. I should have protected her, my baby. Stopped her from seeing him. Never allowed it all. I just didn't think he would do it again.'

Things were different when Mum was a girl. It was the sixties and her whole family would have been classed as outcasts, destroyed, that's if they believed her at all, if they hadn't swept it under the carpet. There was no support for victims and sexual abuse was taboo – to think about it, to talk about it, to acknowledge it went on.

It wasn't going to be easy to convince a court that a woman who'd been abused by a man when she was a child would allow her own child to have contact with him. It's clear-cut to people who haven't been abused, who don't understand.

It was a gritty court case. Jemima had to give evidence. Her grandfather was found guilty. He was given four years in prison. Mum and daughter both went for counselling. Jemima eventually took the ring off.

Who's lying?

Our unit was staffed with six officers. All work and no play made for a dull team and a difficult caseload. We made sure that every couple of weeks or so we'd go out for at least an hour together after work to relax, cast off the shrouds and release any tension. We agreed not to discuss work and to switch off.

This was far from the times when I'd be going for a drink after work every day or when some CID officers would imbibe in the local hostelry for a bit of lunchtime liquid refreshment. The Gene Hunt days were long gone.

We did know how to have a laugh, though. One Friday night turned into an impromptu few hours and we decided to play a game. We had to say three things about ourselves that nobody in the group knew and only one of the things could be false. Every time someone guessed the wrong truth, they'd have to take a swig of whatever they were drinking.

There were some crackers told by those scoundrel police officers. The delivery of some of the lies was so convincing.

One DC said his father used to be a professional footballer back in the 1970s.

Another said he had written a book on rare birds found on the Farne Islands.

Someone else said she was related to Mary Queen of Scots and could prove it.

Another said he slept with a teddy he'd had from birth and couldn't go anywhere without it. We believed him!

Another said his real name was Ignatius Pratt but he'd changed it when he joined the job.

Here are my three:

Before joining the Met, I almost became a nun with the Diocese of Durham. (To convince them of this I reeled off the books of both the Old and New Testament.)

I had my first tattoo, a tiny red scorpion at the top of my left thigh, at the age of thirty-two.

I once went skiing on my own and the airline lost all my luggage. On the first day I dislocated my knee falling down the piste. A family with three boys, also on holiday, decided to look after me. I ended up being their unpaid nanny for the fortnight.

Can you guess the lie?

The man in the corner

I saw his reflection behind the glass front door. It was like he was standing there waiting for us. I knocked twice. He opened up, bent over a stick, wizened and feigning helplessness. To anybody else, he was a sick old man to be pitied. To us, he was a suspected paedophile and he fitted the cliché perfectly.

Gordon Fletcher's apparent surprise and protestations meant nothing but we were still polite. We had to make sure we did nothing to make him aggressive or to aggravate the situation. Keep on his better side and there was more of a chance he would speak, or perhaps confess. Make him annoyed or angry and we'd lose him. I could have gained my Equity card the amount of times I've been pleasantly polite to paedophiles.

We searched the cluttered home while trying not to breathe in too deeply. Stale smoke and cloying heat stuck to my clothes like the strongest adhesive.

We searched for over an hour until we found our evidence.

On the unclean windowsill in the upstairs toilet stood a tree-shaped air freshener. It claimed to be Fresh Pine but it was far from fresh and any scent had long gone. The six-year-old girl

I had interviewed the previous day described it in detail, including the broken knot on the thread which accounted for why it was propped up instead of hanging down. This proved she had been upstairs in his house and in his toilet. I recalled her describing the things he'd made her do and how she said she felt sick as she remembered them when telling us.

We found the suitcase in the corner of the spare bedroom, fawn and battered with two sprung metal clasps. It contained a bundle of yellowing newspapers. Gordon Fletcher said it held every article relating to his deceased hero nephew.

The seven-year-old boy our man had allegedly been abusing for months told us the man with the walking stick and terrible cough had shown them to him inside the house the first time anything happened between them.

Mr Fletcher had a single bed three mattresses high in his bedroom. It was adorned with an orange candlewick bedspread. My nan had had one of those, exactly the same, on the bed I slept in when I stayed at her house as a child. The memory of it stuck with me while I searched the room. Gordon Fletcher sat in the corner watching me with sharp needle eyes, a tut escaping now and again from his otherwise tight lips.

A five-year-old girl in her video interview described in detail how she'd plucked strands from the cover when they were both underneath it and he was doing things to her. I had plucked strands from my nan's candlewick bedspread but I had done it in innocence. Another memory soiled as I found the pockmarks where threads had been pulled, little holes freshly puckered.

In the downstairs lounge in the old cupboard, right at the back behind crust-topped bottles of spirits, we found scrapbooks full of children cut out from catalogues, their heads stuck onto the bare bodies of voluptuous women and naked men. And the other way round too, children's bodies with heads of adults. The officer with me balked. Unfortunately, these books didn't prove anything. It wasn't against the law, back then, to do such things. But I knew what it meant. This old man was not an innocent man. Many paedophiles had similar homemade collections.

We pored over every inch of his house. The scenes of crime officers came to photograph everything we found that we considered evidence. Still, he sat, Gordon Fletcher, watching and rocking in the corner of the room. None of it was conclusive evidence and we had yet to hear his version of events. I knew he would have excuses. He would be a tough nut because you don't get to over seventy and conviction-free as a paedophile without being wily. Or innocent. It wasn't often a 73-year-old man with no previous convictions was arrested for child abuse. There were plenty of them, I have no doubt, but we rarely had the chance to catch up with them at that age.

At the station the police doctor came to assess Mr Fletcher. He asked for his solicitor, too. His medication was brought to the station by weeping relatives. Not one of his three daughters called to ask after him.

By six o'clock that night we were ready to interview Gordon Fletcher.

His denials were swift, his answers florid. 'They're all little sluts, making up stories to get me into trouble. I'm an old man who hasn't had sex with anyone for years, never mind with children. What do you think I am?'

I didn't reply.

'Of course that six-year-old has been in my toilet. She knocked on my door, crying to be let in for a wee. What was I to do?' He started a coughing fit. 'I'm a kind old man who gives kids sweets and stuff,' he cried.

He didn't answer when I asked him, 'What stuff?'

'Yes, that boy has seen my suitcase. I often have it out on the front step, looking through it. All the kids like to see my suitcase. My nephew is a local hero and he meant a lot to me. Now he's dead, killed in the war that's not even ours.'

His tears flowed and we had to allow it. Tears of self-pity, not grief.

'That five-year-old is always in my garden, sneaking in to play. I had my bedspread on the washing line and I caught her pulling it apart, the little rascal. I'll bloody bray her for it the next time, causing me all this trouble,' he said.

'She described your bedroom perfectly.'

'She's mistaken. I've just changed my room around, got new furniture. There's no way she would know what's in the room. The television is from downstairs. I only put it there two days ago,' he said.

I pointed out I had video interviewed her three days before and it recorded not only her words but her emotion, things and feelings that most five-year-olds would have no concept of. 'She said you made her watch a rude film with naked people in it and while it was on the screen, you were doing things to yourself and told her you would keep her warm in the bed.'

He said, 'She told you wrong.'

I described in detail the things she had said.

'I usually fall asleep in the chair in the corner of the room while watching documentaries, history, war programmes. Not porn.' He insisted she was lying.

We saved the best until last. We had the photographs taken by SOCO. When we had lifted the television from the top of the dresser in the bedroom there was a layer of thick dust, evidence the TV hadn't been moved in weeks, if not months. The porn film was still inside the video hatch. It was no documentary.

When we put it to him, it was then he feigned a heart attack.

Today he walks without his stick and he's developed a cleaning obsession. Three years inside the pokey does that to a paedophile.

Head case

It wasn't all doom and gloom. There were opportunities for lighter moments, glimmers of hope in a sometimes dark and depressing world.

Although always busy with a high caseload, we hadn't had a referral for nearly a week. It was most unusual and almost unheard of. I suppose that's why I decided to go with social services on a joint investigation when we otherwise might have left it up to them to make the initial assessment.

The allegation seemed straightforward enough. A school had contacted social services to report a six-year-old boy with deep dark bruising on his forehead. When asked by his teacher what had happened, he said, 'Me mam did it, Miss. Last night.'

A strategy meeting, where multi-agency professionals get together to make a plan of action, had been held mid-afternoon. The family were an open case to social services as a family in need of some help. Mum was a single parent with five children and she was struggling to cope. She had a child with special needs and her parents had recently been killed in a car accident on holiday so she had no support. A family resource worker was helping her and the children, and they had been doing well. There were no previous child protection concerns.

We agreed that we would do this as a joint investigation and I was to go to the school with the social worker to see the boy. The team manager rang the school to ask them to contact the mum to meet us in the head teacher's office just before home time.

When we arrived at the school the head teacher told us mum had refused to come to school as she was too busy with her younger children. The message was, if we wanted to speak to her we would have to go to her.

By the time this was relayed, the classroom assistant had allowed Alfie, the young boy with the bruise, to go with his mum's friend who usually collected him on Thursdays.

In child protection matters, the welfare of the child is paramount. Where there is an allegation of harm, the agencies must make an assessment as to what risk the alleged perpetrator is to children. If a child makes an allegation of assault against his mum and is then allowed to go home, the risk of further injury is high, so of course we were a little worried.

The family home was two streets away. Pam, the social worker, and I, rushed around to the address, arriving at the same time as little Alfie and his mum's friend, who had stopped for a blether at the school gates.

'Alfie, get in here,' shouted his mum, Kelly, when she saw us.

Alfie scampered into the house without giving us a glance, bounding in to chaos and happy to do so. He didn't look frightened or scared, which was a positive sign. Or maybe not. Perhaps he was so used to being hit or hurt that he didn't flinch and accepted a beating as part of normal family life. It was hard to call it straight off.

Kelly Mills stood in the doorway. 'What do you want?'

She looked harassed. A toddler wearing a T-shirt and nappy was hanging off her legs and crying. A far too loud television boomed out from the living room. A child's voice shouted from upstairs, 'Mam, mam. Maaaaaaam! She's got me Game Boy and she won't give it to meeeee!'

We introduced ourselves and asked if we could go inside.

'What for? Will it take long? I'm busy, what with the kids and getting their tea. Is summat wrong?'

As we walked through to the living room I was mentally working out the logistics if we had to take all five children into care.

'I hope not,' I said. 'We've come because we've received information that Alfie has a large bruise on his forehead. We've had to call to find out what happened.'

'What? My Alfie? Did he do it at school?' Kelly picked up the toddler at her feet and swung him onto her hip. She picked up a dummy from the floor, plugged it into the little one's mouth and shush-shushed him. 'Is he okay? They never said.' She shouted, 'Alfie! Alfie! Come 'ere, son!'

It was all back to front and not how we'd normally do things. 'No. Not at school. Do you mind if we talk to him? On his own for a few minutes?' We needed to know from him, without any influence, how he came by a bruise.

'Did a teacher do it? Is that why they wanted me to go to school? Oh my god! A teacher hit him? Alfie!'

'No! No. Not a teacher,' I said. This was going wrong by the second.

Then it dawned on her. Kelly looked at me, open mouthed, and tried to speak but nothing came out. Then she stuttered, 'Me? You mean me? You think I hit him? You're joking? He can be a little bastard sometimes but I don't hit me kids. Alfie! Alfie? Get here now, son. Now!'

He popped up by her side, poking his head around her waist, full of big grins and mischief. 'What, Mam?'

'Hi, Alfie,' I said smiling at him. 'My name is Ash. I'm a police lady.'

385

He blinked at me.

Pam said, 'Hi. I'm Pam and I'm a social worker. I work with Ash.'

'Can I 'ave a biscuit, Mam?' he asked, pulling at his little brother's legs.

'No you can't. Tea's in a bit. What's this about you've got a bruise on your head?' Kelly put the toddler onto the floor, prompting him to cry again. She grabbed hold of Alfie's head and pulled at his blond hair, searching for something, anything, that might indicate a bruise or mark.

Pam piped up, 'It's on his forehead.'

Kelly smudged her son's floppy fringe out of his eyes and there was clearly a dark mark across the length of his forehead, black, purple and a whole range of mixed dark colours. Kelly laughed. 'That? You mean that?' She howled. 'Oh my bloody good god. I don't believe it. You came here because o' that?'

I looked at Pam. She looked at me. We were confused.

'Did that bloody school tell ya I did it? You bloody idiots!'

Pam said, 'Well . . . yes . . . they made the referral. Can I take a look, please?'

'Come with me. Both of ya.' Kelly dragged Alfie by his hand into the kitchen. Pam and I followed. Kelly picked up a raggy tea towel and ran it quickly under the tap. She wiped it across Alfie's forehead, taking with it a huge black streak, smudging colours across her son's forehead. 'Alfie, did you tell ya teacher I did that?' She poked his brow.

'Yes, Mam. She asked me how I got it and I told her. I said you did it last night, Mam. Can I have a biscuit now? Please?'

Kelly turned back to us. 'See? Yes, I did it. Last night. It was Halloween! I got the kids dressed up and put make-up on them. Alfie wanted to be a Frankenstein Zombie thing. It was late when we came home so I asked them to wash their faces themselves while I sorted out the little 'uns. I didn't notice Alfie hadn't washed his head, did I? It's bloody face paint, you morons.'

Morons. I guess that was deserved, if a bit unfair for it to be directed at us. The teacher, maybe . . . but I knew where mum was coming from.

'That's fine, Kelly. Absolutely fine. Great! We have to check out all referrals and we're just doing our jobs. No problem, not a problem at all, we're glad it wasn't anything more. No harm done . . .' etc, etc, etc.

Yes, we did feel like idiots. No, I couldn't argue when Kelly asked us to leave. Yes, I understood that she was a bit peeved.

'I asked you lot for help. And you come in here and accuse me of hurting me kids? And I'll be having words with that school an' all. How come they can't tell the difference between a bruise and face paint?' She may have added a swear word or two into the mix but I wasn't going to challenge her. She had a point.

On the way back to the office, Pam and I had to laugh. If only the teacher had investigated a bit further. If only all cases were as simple to solve. Better face paint than a bruise any day. The reality was, it would have been tragic if the allegation of assault was true. It's much better to able to laugh than to cry at the end of the day. And that's the rub of our work.

When the Twin Towers fell

It started off as an ordinary day. If you're the sort of police officer who doesn't care too much about people, someone who cares more about arrest figures, then I suppose it would be a good day. But I'm not that sort of person. Taking away someone's liberty is a big deal and whenever someone is arrested they remember it for ever, except perhaps the junkies or the drunks.

It isn't always necessary to bust down a door at six o'clock in the morning. Often when people know the police are looking for them they contact the station themselves. When Andrew Banks phoned my office wanting to know when I would be calling to arrest him, I made an appointment for him at twelve o'clock on 11 September. He arrived, complete with solicitor, at a quarter to the hour. He was understandably nervous and a bit upset. Even though he knew why we needed to interview him, he cried when I said we'd received an allegation that he'd abused his twelve-year-old granddaughter, Abigail, and I arrested and cautioned him.

When we interviewed him, his old wrinkled hands shook. I noticed his smart fingernails, his polished shoes, his shirt and tie. Like a gentleman, he'd dressed for the interview. He could barely speak, stuttering over each word he tried to get out. He denied any wrongdoing and insisted he loved his granddaughter but she had been mistaken. He didn't call her a liar or discredit her. He didn't say anything bad about her at all.

When he asked for a drink of water we stopped the interview. There was a tiny kitchen in the custody office, no bigger than a cupboard, and I made up cups of instant tea that came with the sugar added whether you wanted it or not. I figured Mr Banks wouldn't complain.

The custody gaoler poked her head into the room and said, 'Have you heard?'

'Heard what?' I'd been in the interview for over an hour so the chance of hearing anything that day was slim.

'The Twin Towers . . . a plane . . .' She shook her head. 'It's just been on the radio. A plane's crashed into one of the Twin Towers . . .'

'What?' I didn't really comprehend what she was saying. 'How?'

'Dunno. People are jumping out of the building, out of the windows, trying to escape the fire, the collapse . . .'

I thought it was a dreadful accident. All those poor people on the plane and those in the building. It sounded terrible.

I returned to the interview room with plastic cups of fake tea and focused on the man I knew wasn't going to confess any crime.

We concluded forty minutes later. Mr Banks was given bail to return to the police station in a few weeks' time so we could make further enquiries. By the time he left our custody, the world knew of the most horrific terrorist attack to befall New York. For the rest of the day everyone was glued to the news as it unfolded, unable to concentrate or work on anything. It was an unforgettable and memorable day and a tragedy beyond belief.

A few days later I re-interviewed Mr Banks's granddaughter. Her cheeks burned red and she hung her head.

'I'm sorry. I think it was a dream. I'd been watching *EastEnders*. Someone was abused and I dreamt it happened to me. I told my friend who told her mam who told my mam and I thought I'd be in trouble if I said it didn't happen because I had said it did, but I was really dreaming.' It came out in a gabble, fast and furious. 'It just got worse and worse and I didn't think you'd really arrest my granddad.'

She sobbed in her mother's arms and her mother sobbed too.

I was as sure as I could be that she'd made it up. When I'd first interviewed her I'd had my doubts about the vague recollections and insubstantial evidence but we'd still had to take her seriously and investigate properly.

I paid a visit to Mr Banks and told him we were compelled to investigate every allegation and in this case we were pleased to inform him there would be no further action. This was the end of it, case closed.

The poor man. 'It's okay. I forgive her,' he said. 'She's my grand-daughter. She didn't realise what she was saying. Not really.'

The unshed tears in his eyes shone with sadness and shame and I knew he would forgive her. For a while things would be difficult for the family but they'd find a way through.

I'll never forget the day the Twin Towers fell. And neither will Andrew Banks.

Bin-bag kids

I knew we'd get the call one day. You hope it won't come but when someone answers the phone, takes the message and all the while looks you in the eye, you know it's one of those times.

I picked up my suit jacket from the back of my chair, applied a sliver of lipstick, and ran a brush through my hair. Twenty-three Romaine Crescent, up on the Manor Bridge estate. I knew the address. It was one on the list, the long list of those in my head that I'd hoped we'd never have to revisit, but of course, we usually did.

I took the new girl on the team, DC Sarah Fletcher. She'd had five years in the job and although she'd seen the obligatory amount of dead bodies and dealt with the usual number of investigations, nothing quite prepares you for one like this.

'Did you pick up the file?' I asked her.

'Yes,' she said. 'It's in my briefcase. What's the new evidence?'

I navigated the new roundabout by the superstore supermarket. 'It's not new evidence. It's the same as it ever was. Only, it's finished now.'

'Is it a molesting case?'

She obviously hadn't read the file. 'There's all sorts of reasons we get involved in these families. If you scan the file, you'll get the gist of it.'

She flicked open the buff-coloured case file. She looked at the photos, which were blurred and old and showed circular bruising on the back of a young child. That was the first case we were involved in with little Kelvin Grainger. His mother took the rap for that and I always wondered if it had really been his old man, Big Kelvin.

'Mum got a suspended sentence,' I told Sarah as she turned the photos to the side and picked up another blue binder. Another set of SOCO photographs. This time the boy looked about five and sported a reddish-purple black eye, a split lip and a mark on his chin. 'We couldn't proceed on that one. They said he'd fallen off his bike. The doctors wouldn't say otherwise, though everyone suspected something else.'

'Why was he allowed to stay?' Sarah asked.

'It's not as black and white as that. It's frustrating at times but procedures are that families should stay together wherever possible. You have to look at the bigger picture and that's where all the other agencies come in. The first time, when he was two, mum was pregnant. She said she found it difficult to cope. Big Kelvin was on and off the scene, getting into bar brawls, heavily into drugs and about to get sent down for dealing and handling stolen goods. He was looking after some knock-off gear for his brother who was already inside. And even though it was never reported, everyone knew he and her were fighters. Never any domestic violence reports but she often had a black eye, or twist burns up her arm. Social services said they could work with the family and Kelvin was put on the child protection register.'

I could see Sarah digesting all this information as she scanned the reports and case file.

'Big Kelvin used it as mitigation for a lenient sentence in his court case. He played on the need to protect his missus and kids, said he had to look after them because she was so stressed with the child protection issues and postnatal depression. He never got sent down. Not then.'

I remembered the family well. I'd dealt with all four previous child protection cases involving Kelvin and his baby brother Clarke. I'd taken them into foster care when their mother left. She just disappeared one day leaving them home alone. Big Kelvin was inside doing a five-year stretch for dealing cocaine. He did well inside and got early release. He came out to get his boys back, and to be fair he seemed to be doing a good job. He told Claire, the social worker, he intended to keep on the right road and bring up his sons like a decent father. When I saw him at the last case conference he looked quite smart in his jeans and suit jacket, white T-shirt and black loafers. He'd slathered on too much Lynx, but you can't fault him for that. Little Kelvin had settled back into his old school and the baby wasn't a baby anymore. He was nearly four and had a place at a local private nursery, funded by social services, and he was just the sort of kid who would benefit most.

It was one of those cases you hoped, really hoped, would be a success story. One of those houses you never get called back to. But you know it's always there, that the possibility exists.

I pulled up outside 23 Romaine Crescent, parking behind the redundant ambulance and the police patrol car on the corner. I was back into the world of little Kelvin Grainger.

'Okay, Sarah?' I asked. 'You ready for this?'

'Yes,' she whispered.

I could see her set her jaw, a tiny change to her face, teeth clenched. She pulled her jacket close to her chest and stamped her feet to un-crease her trousers. I reached into the back of the car for my overcoat. The air had a nip in it. I spied the roll of black bags on the back seat. I knew we would need them. I reached in and slid the roll into my handbag. I took out a packet of chewing gum. I'd probably need that too.

'Stick of chewing gum, Sarah?' I offered.

'No thanks,' she said.

She'd learn. I shut the car door and snapped the lock shut.

The row of eerily quiet houses belied the presence of curtain-twitchers, who I knew would be watching, jungle drums banging. Police weren't strangers around here.

I walked up the path to the house. In one corner, beneath a hedge, I saw a bunch of snowdrops, hanging like sorrowful mourners. They looked beautiful. I had the urge to grab them up, tie them together and lay them at the door. I knew what I was going to have to do wasn't going to be pleasant. I just wanted something nice to help make it better. I placed a foot on the front step of the house and a stench of stale smoke hit me. These houses always had the heating on full and the warmth mingled with the aroma of dirt and fags making my stomach turn. I felt my morning toast rise and forced it down, my digestion sturdier and more accustomed these days.

Anticipation was a pig in cases like this. The sooner we went inside, the better for everyone. I was aware of Sarah's breath on the back of my neck and could tell by her rapid breathing that she was nervous. I wanted to tell her, it never goes away, that feeling, that dread, you just get used it. It sticks to every strand of your hair, every inch of your clothing, forever there.

I took a step. And another. I was in the front room. I saw his body, lying there, badly dehydrated and tangled up in a ripped and dirty sleeping bag on top of the grubby settee, a heroin stick hanging from a vein in his arm. A lifeline taut with a tourniquet, a drop of blood on his bare arm. His body was slumped, not pumping with life anymore. Big Kelvin Grainger, the daddy.

No doubt it was an accidental overdose. It happens all the time. They come off the drugs. They do well, are clean for a while, make the right noises and make the right effort. But temptation is too much. They mix with the same crowd and the invitations are there. I could see it all around the room. A boy's card night. A toke or two. A hit. So he takes the stick offered and the quantity is too much. His body has cleared it out of his system and it's fatal. Complete.

A uniformed officer came into the room from the adjoining kitchen. 'SOCO's been. We're about done here. Just waiting for the undertaker to collect the body to go to the mortuary.'

'Right,' I acknowledged. 'Where are the kids?'

'Over the road with a woman called . . .' – he checked his notebook – 'Debbie Smith, number thirty-six.'

I knew her. She was a nosy neighbourly sort who would be glad to take the kids in. For an hour or two. She could say she was there, that she helped, and she would try to find out all the gossip, want to be the local hero.

I took in the scene. A fold-up table in front of the settee, two packs of playing cards, one red- and one blue-backed, scattered across the table, some on the floor. An empty bottle of vodka, a litre bottle of cheap corner-shop cola, an overflowing ashtray of fag ends and reefers, half-a-dozen empty and crumpled-up tins of strong lager. And the leftovers of a couple of kebabs, torn and bitten pitta breads with smears of congealing chilli sauce.

'I thought he'd given up the drugs,' I said more to myself than anyone else. Disappointment hit me hard in the chest. I'd hoped it would be different, for little Kelvin, at least. There was hope, once. I turned to Sarah. She was pale, standing there, clutching her briefcase as if afraid to put it down on the floor, the sticky carpet with dog hairs and debris. I glanced down and doubted the carpet had seen a vacuum cleaner in weeks, if not months.

I looked at Sarah, feeling sympathy for her on this her first bin-bag kid case. 'We'll wait until the body has been collected then we'll sort out the kids. Will you phone Claire, the social worker, please? Let her know we're here waiting at the address and won't bring the boys over until dad's body has gone. We'll sort out some stuff for them. I doubt there's much. Only a couple of bin bags full. I don't think they have much in the way of clothes or toys.'

I glanced around, saw some photos on the mantelpiece and made a mental note to put them in a bag. How awful it was taking kids into care, their worldly possessions held in bin bags as they are taken into social services offices awaiting transportation to another life. A tragedy, lives ruined, kids who deserved better. There was a chance for Clarke. He was young enough and hadn't been through as much. But Kelvin. I'll always have a soft spot for Kelvin. Such a cheeky boy with a dimpled grin. How could he ever forget the day he found his dad dead with a heroin stick in his arm?

Pets at home

They say never work with children or animals. Sometimes you don't have any choice.

When the social worker, Tracey, and I called on the Pinder family they didn't know we were coming. I'd like to think they'd have tidied up if they had but I have a feeling it wouldn't have made any difference. It was one of those ramshackle houses that you think might be quaint and cosy inside if it wasn't for the cobwebs stuck fast with time and grime, creeping up the inside of the windows to the corners. Or the old faded brasses adorning the walls, the dried-up flowers wilting in drought-stricken vases, peeling wallpaper and crumbling paint that had long ago given up the shabby-chic look.

Mrs Pinder was a tiny Scottish woman with long grey hair. She wore half-moon glasses that were forever falling down. To say she was scrawny would be unkind but accurate. She welcomed us in. 'Come in. Mind the step. I'll make some tea.' She beckoned us into her house. 'It's a dreich day out there today.'

An unclean waft of sweat and heat emanated from the front room, cloying, wrapping itself around us.

'No tea for me, thanks,' I said. I'd long ago given up accepting tea and other offers of hospitality from most of the houses we visited.

Mrs Pinder had no fat on her; she was almost anorexic. Mr Pinder was no Jack Sprat. He sat in the corner of the room in a recliner, his fleshy arms hanging limp over the sides of the chair, his frame taking up a quarter of the room. His large feet lay exposed, propped up on a fake fur pouffe. His big toes were incredibly hairy.

Mrs Pinder said, 'Nae bother. Tea never goes amiss.' She moved across the room to the Aga-style cooker that stood against the back wall of the small lounge-cum-kitchen and lifted the lid from the large silver kettle. She peered inside like a witch watching a cauldron bubble. Her glasses steamed up and fell down. 'A couple a minutes more,' she said.

I envisaged frogs legs and bay leaves swirling in the water. 'We've come about your report to Childline, Mrs Pinder.' With a mixture of horror and bemusement, my eyes were again drawn to Mr Pinder's feet. I had to stop myself staring.

'The children will be home at half past three. I'm glad you've come, I'd rather talk to you without them here.' She waved us to a two-seater settee nestled in the bay window. It was covered with magazines, knitting and a bundle of cats. 'Take a seat,' she said.

Tracey had no hesitation in sweeping the sleeping animals to the floor.

I shoved last month's TV mag and assorted newspapers into the back of the settee and sat down, almost kicking the sleeping black dog by my feet. A bird squawked in my right ear and I turned to see a parakeet in a cage, its floor covered in bird poop. It was parallel to my head height and I wondered how I'd missed seeing it. The bird squawked again.

'What have you got to tell us, Mrs Pinder?' I asked, opening up my statement folder, pen poised.

Mr Pinder replied, 'Oh, she's got a lot to tell. All about that bloke who lives on the corner. Kids going in his house all times o' day and night. He's one of them, he is, an' then some.'

'Mrs Pinder?' I turned to his wife.

'Oh yes, Mac's right. I see him, encouraging the kids into his house. Sweets, money, computer games, all that sort of stuff. He's dodgy, you ask me.'

'How do you know?'

'I see him. Watch him from that window, I do.' She pointed to the bay behind me. 'Always kids hanging about his house. The teenagers go to him for fags. He buys 'em for 'em. And porn! Gives 'em it for nowt to start with then charges 'em, adding a few bob on top for his bother. Bear-baiting, that's what he's doing.' She stirred the large kettle with a wooden spoon.

Tracey asked, 'Do you know the kids? Who they are? Where they live?'

'All the local kids go there. Everyone round here knows it but daren't speak up. They're 'fraid of him. Ex-army bloke, big baldy heid, bull-frog eyes. Nasty piece o' work. Made old Mr Talbot take down their adjoining fence and I ken he was the one who—'

A huge commotion of squealing and screeching erupted from somewhere at the back of the house

'Just the guinea pigs rutting for their food,' she said, waving the spoon in the air. 'I'll have to feed them in a minute. And the mice and rats. We got two degus yesterday. Funny little creatures they are.'

As if by magic, summonsed by her wooden wand, three gerbils ran out from beneath the settee. They ran across my shoes, up the fur pouffe and onto Mr Pinder, climbing up his legs. One nibbled at the hard skin on his bare feet. He smiled.

I lifted my feet off the grubby floor and shuffled a few inches across the settee towards Tracey.

Mr Pinder said, 'It's okay. They're my pets. Come for a snack.' He made some tutting noises and sucked in saliva between his tiny rodent-like teeth. He produced a handful of seeds from a pouch hanging down from the arm of his chair. A gerbil ran up to his chest and he fed it a dried kernel of sweetcorn.

I attempted to take a deep breath but the air was thick and too warm. I felt giddy. I shrugged out of my jacket and folded it onto my lap. I watched, mesmerised, as the gerbils played with the man in the chair, their little claws denting his flesh as they ran. He seemed to be enjoying it.

Mrs Pinder poured hot water from the kettle into a fat brown teapot. She plonked a hand-knitted tea cosy on top. The way she rattled the teacups and saucers, it was no wonder they were chipped.

I knew I needed to get out of there when a gerbil started sucking at one of Jack Pinder's toes.

'Do you know the guy's name?' asked Tracey, trying but failing not to look at the foot-fetish gerbil.

Pinder replied, 'Oh yes. Richard Hart. The kids call him Braveheart. Or Dick Heart.' She pursed her lips and nodded, as if we understood, knowing.

I made rushed notes, not sure if I'd be able to read them back, but I didn't care. I felt the burn at the back of my throat. It was sore.

A grey fluffy cat sleeping next to the dog stood up. I might have thought it cute in a different house. It lifted its tail high, farted, licked its bottom, then jumped onto my lap.

I shot up, brushing the poor animal off me. 'Urgh, furgh, fluff, furrah, pah!' Something like that. I like animals, I really do, but a bit like kids, I prefer my own. 'Sorry. Sorry,' I said, sitting down, a flurry of hand movements brushing a zillion grey cat hairs from my trousers.

When I looked up, Mr and Mrs Pinder were looking at me with such disappointed faces: down-turned mouths and wide eyes.

I lied. 'Sorry. I'm a bit allergic. Please forgive me.'

'Oh!' said Mr Pinder, looking at his wife. 'In that case love, give her an antihistamine.' He turned to me. 'We keep them especially for visitors. Surprising the amount of people who have fur allergies.'

'No!' I shouted, holding up a hand like a traffic cop. 'Nope. It's okay. Really. We won't be much longer.' I ran a finger around the inside of my collar. I was very hot.

I knew Tracey could sense my discomfort in the way that you get to know the people you work with, begin to know how they think. A bit like a marriage. After all, it was a partnership.

'I think that's all we need for now,' she said, looking down at her scribbling. 'I can smell your dinner cooking, so we'll be off. We've got your phone number if we need anything else.'

'But what about your cup of tea?' said Mrs Pinder. 'And I've not started on the dinner yet.' She looked at us. She sniffed.

I sniffed.

Tracey sniffed.

Mr Pinder sniffed.

I could smell something. Tasty. A bit like chicken.

Mrs Pinder's arms shot up like she was surrendering, about to be shot. Her hands clasped over her mouth. She stood wide-eyed. Her glasses fell off as she scrabbled for a tea towel. She rushed over to the Aga-style cooker and flung open the oven door. She pulled out a bundle. Her wails echoed around the room. I'll never forget the distress of that poor woman as she flung it onto the work surface.

Mr Pinder howled like an injured wolf. He struggled to get out of his reclining chair and failed. 'Noooooo!' It was pitiful.

I looked at the table, at the charred shell. I looked at Tracey. It was really horrible, truly terrible. It was smoky black. It was smelly. It was a tortoise. It was darkly hilarious and deeply distressing all at once. I had to stop myself from being sick. And from laughing. I didn't know what to do. It wasn't funny. It was bad. Horrid.

Mrs Pinder sobbed. 'Angus! Angus! Oh, it's my fault! He was so cold this morning! I put him in the oven to warm up a bit. I forgot him! He's cooked!'

I gagged. I saw Tracey gag. Mr Pinder collapsed into a faint in his chair. It cracked. Or maybe it was his heart breaking.

Mrs Pinder ran to the sink with Angus in the tea towel. She turned on the tap and water sprayed everywhere, stinging cold drops bouncing off every surface.

It was too late. Angus was gone.

It was time to leave. We backed out of the house slowly, a mark of respect, heads bowed, necks buried in our collars . . .

For Stan, Santa

I hadn't expected Stan to be indoors as it was benefit day, the last before Christmas. I knocked on the front door and the cheap hollow wood echoed back.

Stan opened the door to me. 'Come in, thanks for coming.' He was gruff and unshaven and I saw signs of weariness and despair etched into the lines of his face. The young boy by his feet grabbed Stan's legs tight.

I stepped into the house and noted a tatty couch and a solitary armchair. On a shelf in the alcove sat a portable television with the obligatory wire hanger for an aerial. It would be Christmas in three days but this house showed no signs of it.

'How can I help?' I asked. People didn't usually call child protection unless they had to. Especially at Christmas.

Stan looked at me and all I saw was hopelessness and defeat. Once a drug addict, a thief, a petty criminal, today he was trying to be a responsible father. 'She wants him for Christmas.'

I had an image of his little boy, Tom, stuffed with a ribbon around his neck and presented to his drug-addicted, alcohol-riddled mother.

'She said it was her rights . . . but she's back on the crack . . . and I can't do it. I can't let him go.'

'No, of course not. You mustn't. What are your plans?'

'I don't have any. I've borrowed a telly from a mate.' He pointed to the small screen in the corner. 'I've got twenty quid for some shopping. I'm gonna cook a dinner. For me and Tommy. A chicken if I can get one tomorrow. I'll get him some chocolate and stuff. Treats, whatever I can afford.'

I bent down to the little boy pulling at my legs. 'Hiya, mate.'

I picked him up and he smiled. Tommy was small for three. I remembered when I took him away from his mother in the maternity ward after she'd been found jacking up in the hospital grounds an hour after he'd been born. It was one of the most distressing things to see these drug-addicted babies. Stan had looked after Tom ever since, in his 'good enough' way. He'd come off the drugs and kept social services from his door for all but the odd bit of support and cash. An ex-child in care himself, the poor guy had no one but the authorities to help and he hated asking. He tried his best and he loved his son, we all knew that.

'You have the court order, Stan. She can't take him. It's up to you whether you let her in the house to see him but she can't take him if you say no. If there's any trouble, phone 999.'

'Easy for you to say.' He scuffed his shoes on the bare floor, which was uncovered by lifestyle, not design choice.

'I'll speak to social services, make sure Tommy has his children's fund allocation, the presents from the kitty, and I'll ask them if they can sort out a Christmas special bonus payment.' It was the best the local authority could do and I knew he was ashamed to accept it. It wasn't mine to offer but I hoped they would give.

'Thank you,' he said, hands hunched in his pockets, unable to meet my eye.

Of course he was humble. I didn't show I felt his pain. That wouldn't do either of us any good.

For the next two days I thought about Stan and his little boy.

Father and son alone at Christmas, Stan trying to keep on the right side when it would be so easy for him to slip. And there were a few who not only wished it, but expected it.

I wished there was more I could do.

Ten o'clock on the crisp Christmas Eve night, I drove past Stan's house. I parked a few houses up near to the junction. His front room was lit with a string of fairy lights from the pound shop and a couple of wobbly Santas hung from plastic hooks sucked onto the inside of the window.

I saw the upstairs bedroom light flick off. The streets were quiet, the air fresh. I turned off my lights but kept the engine running. I climbed out of the warmth of my little car and opened the boot. I tried not to make a sound as I approached the house. I put a bulging red sack on the step of the terraced house and pounded hard on the door. I rushed back to my car, slammed the door once inside and drove off, no lights, at high speed around the corner.

Stan wouldn't want my charity and hated to ask for help but I was pleased to give it. My kids always had more than enough presents to open and wouldn't miss a few. It would be frowned upon at work so I couldn't mention it. It was wrong to get too involved. Sometimes, though, families stick, and many of us wished there was more we could do. I wasn't God but the least I could to do was play Santa and give Tommy a good Christmas that year.

Chasing motorcycles

As with any posting, you become bogged down with the same old, same old, and it's good to have time out, to step away from the bizarre world you inhabit and step into another, even if it's only for a week, or just one night . . .

In order to raise awareness and recognition of child protection issues we would sometimes deliver training sessions to our uniformed colleagues working at the grittier end. After all, they were the ones who referred cases to us so they needed to know what evidence we needed, and to see that it was more than just a dirty house with children in it.

During one training session a young constable suggested that officers from child protection should go out on patrol with them, be first on scene at these houses, and show them what they should be looking for.

I thought it was a great idea. The bosses weren't so keen but I insisted the PC had a point. If we expected good reporting and correct information, then those at the front end needed to know what was required of them. A couple of lessons at training school isn't enough and it takes time to build up experience. It's no good complaining they haven't done their job or don't know how to fill out a report if nobody has shown them on a practical level what to look for.

That's how I found myself one night duty in the back of a police patrol car.

I squeezed into my musty stab-vest and armed myself with my baton, CS spray and radio. Of course my uniform didn't 'quite' fit after three children, so it was agreed I would wear my own casual clothes. I was looking forward to it, a Saturday night on the run.

The families we dealt with in CPU rarely had intervention on a weekend so it was possible their guard might slip. The multi-agency professionals generally worked Monday–Friday daytime hours, but life continues 24/7 irrespective, and the duty team for out-of-hours cover responded to emergencies only. They also had the whole of the county to cover with maybe only four personnel. With little chance of being caught out, it's understandable for people to relax a little. A lot of our cases came to light because of a call as a result of a domestic, and most domestics occurred on weekends, usually after pub kicking-out time, though it was hard to know what kicking-out time was in a town where many pubs favoured all-hours drinking.

The idea was that our panda unit would aim to deal with the domestics and any calls involving children or sex offences. We would have to respond to other things if needed, so who knows what I might end up dealing with? It felt good to be back at it on the front line.

I was with PC Ian Jefferson, known as Jeff, and the young PC whose idea this thing had been to start with, PC Rory Bacon, whose name still sounds like a spoof.

The shift started off quiet but nobody mentioned the Q word for fear of all hell breaking out. It made no difference, though, because at midnight we were running around chasing our shadows. We'd been to two domestics already but neither had had children present so there was nothing for me specifically to deal with. We then took a report of a missing fourteen-year-old. That was more up my street.

The address was on a private residential housing estate. Town locals called it Sex-in-the-Cityville because of the amount of affluent single mums that lived there. The next estate along was known as Chav-ville because of the number of residents that had been on the *Jeremy Kyle Show*. In fact, all the houses were identical on both estates, but that's judgemental townspeople for you.

Mum met us at the door as we arrived. 'Thank you for coming. I know my Sharmayne is a good girl really but I'm dead worried. She's gone off with a Chav lad. She's only fourteen. Who knows what she's up to?'

We made the obligatory introductions and I said, 'Do you know this lad? Have you tried to contact her?'

'Her mobile went straight to voicemail. She stormed out this afternoon when I saw a love bite on her neck and I knew it was off of him. I told her she wasn't to see him again but she takes not a scrap of notice of me these days. We should never have moved her, but when her dad left we had no choice and she said she wants to go and live with him, but he's got a new girlfriend who doesn't want a sulky teenager hanging around and it's caused all sorts of trouble and my new bloke said that Laurie is a bad 'un, that's him, her boyfriend, Laurie, because he used to go to school with Laurie's dad and now he's in prison and his sister is knocking off the old man next door, and I think he said she might be on drugs and I don't want all that for my Sharmayne because she's a good girl, but she won't do nowt I ask her to do and her dad isn't interested and I'm at my wits end and now she hasn't come home and she'll be pregnant next and I can't—'

'Woah! Stop!' I said, holding up a hand. Sharmayne's mum hadn't taken a breath. I felt exhausted. 'Too much information all at once. Pause a minute. Can we come in?'

'Yes, sorry.' She waved us indoors.

Jeff said he'd wait in the car and write up the last DV report. It didn't need three of us to take details for a Misper (missing person).

Rory was very good at taking down the personal details of Sharmayne, full name, date of birth, hair colour and style, distinctive marks, what she was wearing, all of that stuff.

'Don't forget the love bite on her neck,' said her mum. 'It's underneath her hair, on the left. Or was it the right?'

'How old is Laurie, the boyfriend? And where does he live?' I asked.

'He's seventeen and he lives with his mum and two sisters in Colroy Crescent. Number two, I think. And he has a motorbike.'

'Have you met him?'

'Yes. He's been here a few times. He seems a nice enough boy but he lives on that estate, you know, and you hear all sorts. He's got a job and all that and goes to college, but he's too old for her. And he has a motorbike, did I tell you that?'

It was easy to see Sharmayne's mum was upset. I knew from many other similar cases that it's hard when teenagers strike out and rebel.

'Do you think she's at any risk from him?' I asked.

'Well, no. I don't think so. She's mad for him but I don't think he'll hurt her. But she should have been home by ten o'clock.'

'And you know she's with him?'

'She's always with him. She doesn't see any of her friends anymore. It's always him.'

I had to put it out there because there isn't any gentle way to ask a parent that particular question about their child. In their heads, their almost-but-not-quite grown-up daughter is still a little girl and most won't entertain the notion. 'Do you think she's having sex with him?'

'Oh no! No! Definitely not! I hope not. I don't think so. Well, maybe . . .' and she burst into tears.

It was nearly one o'clock in the morning. I doubted Sharmayne would be anywhere else but with Laurie, but we had to make sure.

'Tell you what, I'll put the kettle on, and PC Bacon will go with the other officer to check out Laurie's address. See if she's there. If she is, they can bring her back.' I nodded to Rory. He looked glad to escape.

I made a cup of my best tea and tried to give Sharmayne's mum my best advice.

'You got teenagers?' she asked me.

'No. Not yet. But I will have. Give it a few years. I have no doubt I'll be tearing my hair out all too soon,' I said.

Cases like this were difficult because social services handed out sex education and condoms and GPs prescribed the pill. Then the police come along and arrest the youth over sixteen and video interview the younger one, when really, seventeen and fourteen, yes it's far too young, yes it's against the law, but it's a consenting act between two people who want to be together. Any force or coercion or drugs or drink and it's a different matter altogether. Then it's rape. But many teenagers, whether parents or society like it, have sexual relations and they have done for many generations before today. This town typically had one of the highest underage pregnancy rates in the whole United Kingdom. It's impractical to police and the best advice can only come from those who accept reality and provide these kids with the tools to deal with it emotionally and practically when their parents don't. In a perfect world. But it isn't a perfect world.

I tried to explain all of this to Sharmayne's mum. She'd calmed down in the twenty minutes it took to drink her tea and for Rory to come back.

'We've been to Laurie's house,' he said. 'She is with him . . . but his mum said they've gone off on his bike somewhere. She thought he was bringing her home. I've got the bike index and it's all registered to him. I've put it out to the other units.'

I had a thought. 'You know, he might have been bringing her back home and maybe he saw the police car outside so they took off again. We know she's with him. We'll see if we can find them. I'll keep in touch and ring you when we pick her up. I'm sure she'll be back in no time.'

I gave her my work mobile number and asked her to ring me if Sharmayne turned up in the meantime. At least everything seemed a lot calmer when we left than when we'd arrived. I climbed back into the panda and asked Jeff if we could have a scoot around the two estates to see if we could catch sight of the couple.

Area searched, no trace.

We then got a call to a domestic on the other side of the ground. It took us the best part of an hour to sort it out. Three children were upstairs, sleeping but not really. I knew the address from previous domestic incidents but they weren't in the system yet. I felt it wouldn't be long before something more serious took place. I told Rory I'd go over the forms with him on refs, which was where we were headed. When we were driving along the high street and almost back at the nick, Jeff piped up, 'Look. The bike. Two's up. What's that index?'

Sure enough, it was Laurie's bike.

Jeff signalled for it to stop. It didn't. The rider throttled the engine and shot off at speed, through a set of lights just changing to red. Jeff switched on the blues and twos and we were off.

We followed him for about a mile but he didn't stop. Rory called for assistance from any other units in the area but drew a blank as everyone was busy. As we approached the maze of a housing estate, the bike suddenly swerved. It drove up onto the kerb and along a public alleyway between two houses. Jeff pulled the panda up to a sharp stop at the side of the dual carriageway.

I opened the rear passenger door and legged it out.

Jeff shouted after me, 'What the hell you doing? You can't run after a motorbike!'

'Watch me,' I yelled back. Okay, they knew a car wouldn't make it through the cut-through but a person could and I didn't give up that easily.

'You'll not catch him,' shouted Jeff.

I ran down the alley and had a choice – left or right?

I picked left. Good choice. There standing by a cooling bike was Sharmayne, pulling off her helmet. Laurie was still astride the bike, panting, adrenalised.

'Hi, guys!' I smiled.

We took a sheepish Sharmayne home and I spoke to mum, promising I'd contact her first thing Monday morning. I suggested mum and daughter had a chat in the meantime. A proper chat, forgetting about chastisement but having a proper discussion about the realities of life and all that it means.

I took Laurie's details and told him to expect a call from me mid-week.

What had he done? Kept his girlfriend out after hours when she pleaded she needed a shoulder to cry on? Yes. Committed any offences? Probably not, but maybe yes. Was it a lesson in child protection? Perhaps. Was it a lesson in life? Yes. We'd found a missing girl and took her home. Did it make a case for CPU to work all hours? Crikey, don't blame me for that!

I loved it all the same, even if I did fall asleep in the back of the panda come five o'clock.

Bad apples

Police officers uphold the law, protect life and property, and come in for a lot of stick for doing so. I know it sounds corny but I joined the police force because I wanted to help people.

As in all professions and in all strata of society, there are those that let the side down. The majority of the people I worked with were decent, hard working and believed in the greater good.

There are people who think the police spend their time stitching people up, fabricating evidence and getting off on the power of the job. I can't deny that people like that exist, but they are rare. And they aren't very well liked. And they don't last long. The rest of us don't want to work with people like that. Why would I want to be associated with someone who was lazy or who didn't treat people well? Not only would it give me a bad name but I'd end up doing all the work. I wouldn't stitch anyone up and as much as I can defend myself in a fight, I'd never start one.

But there are those, that tiny minority, that do.

There was a PC who worked at a station where I was a detective. He would ask for postings as gaoler in the custody office. Two female prisoners alleged he'd indecently assaulted them. One was a drug addict and the other a drunken prostitute. He denied it. They were considered unreliable witnesses.

Late one night I was in the custody office, walking down the cell corridor to speak to a prisoner. One of the doors was open. I looked in as I passed by and I saw the officer with his hand up the skirt of an unconscious woman lying on the stone bench.

I shouted out. 'Hey! What you doing?'

'She's fallen from the bench. I'm just pushing her back up,' he said, straightening her clothing.

I didn't believe him. I told the custody sergeant what I'd seen and he said he'd deal with it, but I knew it was my word against that of the gaoler. The woman was unconscious and totally unaware. There were no independent witnesses.

I knew what I had seen. I was relieved when, a year later, the officer was sacked for an unrelated incident off duty.

Then there was a sergeant who worked with prostitutes. He was sent to prison for living off immoral earnings.

An officer was sacked for having a stolen engine in his car.

A PC was sent to prison for ten years for raping a number of women. Is it any consolation that he was off duty at the time of the attacks?

Two officers, different stations, fifteen years apart, went to jail for murdering their wives.

Three detectives were sacked for giving confidential information from the PNC to criminals.

A PC who was married was sacked for making prostitutes give him sexual favours in the back of the police van in return for not arresting them.

One sergeant was sacked for indecent assault on female prisoners.

Another sergeant, who was known for bullying, was sacked for his inappropriate conduct with female prisoners.

See a pattern?

A female officer was sacked for giving confidential information to her armed-robber boyfriend.

A detective was sacked for giving tabloid newspapers confidential information.

Two constables were sacked for shoplifting and making off when officers tried to arrest them.

An officer was requested to resign for his drug addiction. Another because of his suspicious involvement with drug lords.

There have been police officers sacked and/or sent to prison for downloading child porn.

These people are a minority. I've known hundreds, if not thousands, of police officers. Everywhere has bad apples, rotten to the core, and the police service today is more proactive than ever in pursuing them. The majority of police officers are good, honest, decent, hard working and conscientious. And they do have to bear the sins of their fathers when flawed enquiries and miscarriages of justice are resurrected, such as Hillsborough. It's shameful. I make no excuses for them. But it's not all of us.

Fair cop, guv'nor

The problem I have with crime fiction and TV police drama is the same as most cops. It's just not like that in real life.

To be fair, the last thing I wanted to do when I came home from a hard day on the streets was to read or watch anything to do with the police. Switch the television on and there's a plethora of fly-on-the-wall police programmes. Where's the fun in that? The same with reading misery memoirs. I could write a never-ending series based on the cases I've dealt with.

So what do cops do in their down time? Live their lives like anyone else, I guess. Pre-kids, I read a lot, I socialised a lot, I did a bit of voluntary work and some studying. I look back and wonder, what was it I did do? When I had kids all of my spare time was taken up with being their mum and being involved in their various activities. And doing a degree. I remember never having enough time but it helped me not to dwell on the job. I was far too busy!

Most readers and viewers don't really know how the police work, but it sounds and looks exciting; it's escapism, it's a bit of tense drama or narrative while sitting comfy and safe in your own house. Hence, armchair detectives.

I don't criticise writers of crime fiction. Far from it. There are many credible authors out there who have made a very decent living from writing about death and detectives and dirty deeds. And they certainly don't write their novels with the idea of cops reading them. Now I no longer do the job, I read crime fiction again and watch a bit of detective TV, but I am biased and I am choosy.

Those tired old clichés of coppers should be written out, not in. I know television programmes use police advisors, but I know producers don't always listen and that they go ahead with what they know best – making drama. Maybe real life is not interesting enough and maybe they're right, it's really not. But neither does it happen that a DI and a DC will investigate a serial killer without any other help. Nor will they do the scenes of crime work, or walk into a post-mortem and flick cigar ash into an open chest cavity. Though I do know of a doctor who did that, many years ago.

How many know a sergeant from an inspector from a super-intendent? When do police need a warrant? And when don't they? How would they interview a child witness? And how wouldn't they? How close do officers actually get to their victims and witnesses? Or suspects?

How much of what people read in books or watch on television do they actually believe is true?

If you're considering writing about a cop, or the police generally, you need to do a bit of research and get it right. And for an acknowledgement I'll give you a heads-up.

The waiting room

A lot of police time is spent in hospitals. There are victims of crime to see and doctors and nurses to take statements from. A prisoner may be in need of emergency attention because they've taken an overdose, have been fighting, feigned illness or had a panic attack. Maybe they've been run over.

Perhaps the officer has been injured on duty and is in need of treatment. Or a doctor or nurse has been assaulted. There are those who present at hospital drunk and who become disorderly, meaning the nurses have to call police. Then there are the patients who turn nasty or have relatives that turn up to fight, continuing family feuds in A&E.

I spent many hours at the old Mile End Hospital, The London Hospital (Whitechapel), University College Hospital in central London, St Thomas's, St Mary's, St Clement's and lots more. Many hospitals were grand old buildings, but I had no time for grandiose architecture, however beautiful, because I was too busy sitting with the resident tramps and thieves, trying not to make too much small talk or breathe in too deeply.

I've guarded fourteen-year-old arsonists caught in their own fire, a heroin addict who'd taken a bad toke and died but was resuscitated by emergency staff while his young daughter looked on, and the suspected paedophile who'd tried to hang himself one Christmas after being caught sexually abusing his stepdaughter. There have been breach of the peace suicide attempts that, once in hospital, were no longer a risk. There was the man who wrapped his head in silver foil to stop the voices getting through, and the man who after years of abusing his wife was on the receiving end when she poured a pan of boiling spaghetti over his crotch. One of the saddest was the mother who strangled her young son because his face reminded her of her abusive father. The list is endless. It's no wonder police officers and nurses and doctors develop close professional and personal relationships.

The paramedics have it tough too, working the streets and dealing with the same people the police do. The same goes for social workers. We all deal with the same families, time and again, yet it's the firemen and women who are the only ones that seem to be society's heroes. Everyone loves a fireman. But they see terrible things too. We are all human, fallible and feeling, and all of us who work in these professions are knee-deep in it together.

In my head

When you do a job like policing, you see people at their best and at their worst. The majority of people only come into contact with police in times of distress, so for them everything is heightened: intense passion, fear, guilt, grief, whether as a victim, a witness or a suspect.

When you dip into lives they leave a little of themselves behind and they are there, at almost every turn, these people with their raw emotion.

When I pop into the local supermarket to pick up some shopping, I see them, these ghosts. Three tills ahead, I spy a man. He used to be an advocate for voluntary workers, a person who stood up for people's rights and people's lives. We caught each other's eye. I noticed he was still as sleek as a greyhound, smart and smooth, with fast eyes. We were discreet. We looked away, pretended we hadn't seen, hadn't noticed, didn't know each other.

A few years ago my team raided his house. We took away his computers and those of his wife as she stood and watched, bewildered, wrapping her silky dressing grown around her plump body as we blundered our way through her home. She was a writer and had deadlines but we couldn't rush the job. I wanted her to have her words back but the tech team had many computers to examine and there was a queue. There always is for the worst kind of porn because there's an endless supply of paedophiles with computers to search.

I left the supermarket juggling plastic bags bulging with bread, bananas, coffee and wine. I saw a middle-aged couple walking towards me. They actively tried to avoid me but it was difficult as he had to manoeuvre his crutches.

I'd given him a caution five years ago. I battled with the Crown Prosecution Service because I thought he deserved to be charged, to be taken to court for a decent penalty to be imposed on him for his dirty deeds. Anyone guilty of indecent assault, especially on someone vulnerable like his stepdaughter, deserved more than a slapped wrist. The CPS said not, so he didn't go to court. His name didn't go in the local paper. He didn't work, so he didn't lose his job as many sex offenders do. His wife stood by him rather than her daughter. This wasn't his first time but the rehabilitation of offenders meant his juvenile caution of a similar offence forty years earlier couldn't be brought into it. I challenged the decision but it's called justice, apparently. In my experience, once a paedophile, always a paedophile. They rarely change, if ever. At best, some of them try to control their urges.

I waited until Mr and Mrs Conway hobbled their way past me. I didn't acknowledge them. She was ruddy-cheeked and nagging him. He held his head down. I drove home and locked my front door.

The following day a card was pushed through my letterbox. It was from the Pritchards, a family I'd recently dealt with. The man who was supposed to love and protect them, the husband and father, had instead destroyed them. He was long gone but he'd never be gone. He'd always be there, his presence in their lives. He'd sexually abused the eldest girl ever since she could remember. Her first memory was when she was four years old.

He physically hurt her too. We put him in prison but he won an appeal on a technicality so I can't call him a paedophile. He was now out of prison and running a delivery company, a business I make sure I never use. It was another family I knew too much about and they had sent the card to say thank you for everything, they were grateful for my help even though we didn't get the right result for them. I can't shake them. They know where I live because we live in a small place where everyone knows your name and the colour of your front door.

I put my kids to bed and lay with them for a few moments. I closed my eyes and saw a young boy, Bradley, standing on his doorstep waiting for help to arrive. Not me in particular, but someone, anyone. He called his social worker. He had her mobile number etched in his brain. She was concerned enough to call me. We arrived together, at the same time, and we laughed. It was us again, Cagney and Lacey. Ashley and Tracey. But the laughter didn't reach our eyes.

I climbed from my car as a cider bottle flew past Bradley's ear. It smashed at his feet. His little lips wobbled, as did his stick thin legs. His eyes filled with tears he was too frightened to cry. I ran and grabbed him, held him to me, and shouted into the house.

Chaos ensued. I called my uniform colleagues to help convey Bradley's drunken mother to the station in the back of a police van. I arrested her for neglect, child cruelty and assault on Bradley. It wasn't a specific offence to be a bad parent. Maybe it should be. I took Bradley by the hand and collected some of his possessions. He didn't have many. Another bin-bag kid packed up for foster care.

There was a recipe book in a corner of the rancid kitchen. Bradley wanted to take it because he said he wanted to make cupcakes for his mum when he was allowed to come home again. Despite it all, the neglect and the pain and the vicious words from cruel tongues that should smooth cuts and bruises, these kids still love their abusive parents.

The previous weekend I was at a wedding of some friends. A young waitress, Rachel, served me watery coffee. She was a victim of rape by her uncle and he was now in prison. She looked half-starved and I knew the anorexia she battled with must have returned. She still looked frightened. Haunted. We did what we had to do and pretended we didn't know each other. Some of them prefer it that way.

Every day there is someone, something. Everywhere there are ghosts. I know too much about too many people's lives. I know their names though I sometimes forget, but I always remember their faces. They are there, in my head, forever there.

The end – again

So, here we are. I started at the end and if you've stuck with me, we've come full circle and we are here again. The End.

I hope you've liked my stories. I've kept many light and tried to be humorous because others are dark and definitely not funny. Like life, it's about balance.

I left the police service because my physical health made it impossible to continue. I didn't want to go but I had to as I was classed as having a physical disability. I also had a family to look after and I had to be there for them. I had to be a positive role model, to show them that when life throws a wobbly it's about how you deal with it and move on. It wasn't going to be the end of me, even if it was the end of my career. It's about working with what you've got and what you can do, not moping about what you don't have or can't do. I would still be there doing it now if I could, but in jobs like this, we pay the price. It comes with the job, of course, but at nineteen, or however old you are when you join up, nothing can prepare you for what you will do and see. I chose to do this job and others didn't. Like very many of those that do, we all carry the same-but-different memories.

When I am questioned about my pension, or the issue of pensions is debated in the media, I keep quiet. I turn away and remember. Those of us who have worked in these professions do it because others don't want to or have to. Public sector pensions are good but not that good. And we have earned it.

Since leaving the job, I've changed my life completely. I've gone into a totally different kind of work, one without physical limitations. I got myself a degree and fulfilled a lifetime ambition to start writing. Today I live far, far away from the capital and anywhere else I've policed.

I've been lucky. Policing was my passion, my dream job. To have two dream jobs in one lifetime, I don't know if it's possible, but I'm going to try. I do know nothing will ever beat being in 'the job'.

There are other opportunities. I've had a great time and, yes, I would do it all again. Ian Rankin gave life back to Inspector Rebus so who knows what I can do with Ash Cameron. She isn't done yet.

To you all, cops or otherwise, I leave you with this from my favourite show – *'Let's be careful out there.'*

OTS and other strange things

The police force has its own language. Here are some common acronyms and abbreviations, some of which you may be familiar with. Each force has different policies and procedures, each department its own dialect. Things vary cross-border, cross-county and cross-country.

Armed blagger –	Armed robber
ATS –	Automated traffic system – or traffic lights
Black rat –	Traffic officer
Blagger –	Robber
Blues and twos –	
A body –	An arrested person, or a dead body
Burglary artifice –	Someone pretending to be an official, e.g. gas board, council worker, postman, to gain entry to a house to steal from it
CAD (computer aided despatch) room, control room –	Where the calls and messages are taken and despatched
Civil remedies –	Cases in the civil court that don't end up with criminal convictions and are decided by a judge on the balance of probabilities, if the judge thinks it's more likely to have happened or not, rather than absolutely

sure in criminal cases. Individuals can bring a civil case against another person. A civil case usually doesn't involve the police though they can sometimes be summonsed to attend to state what, if anything, they know or can add.

Clampers –	The wheel clamping van
Clippy, Clip girl, Clip joint –	A place where scantily clad girls would entice men to pay for drinks at extortionate prices and charge them for the pleasure of their company, often with the promise of something sexual taking place, which it rarely did. Men would part with lots of money, by force or desire, and often be left high and dry and broke.
Corres –	Correspondence, admin, paperwork
CPS –	Crown Prosecution Service
CPU –	Child Protection Unit
CRIS –	Crime Reporting and Intelligence System – something the Met implemented in the 1990s – fabulous system despite early teething problems. It holds all intelligence and all reports taken by every officer in the Met policing area. Previously you would have to ring a station to see if they had information about someone or something. Now it's all on the computer and easily accessible to the right people.
CS spray –	Part of the police officer's defence/aid. A canister of 'gas' which is a suspension of particles in a liquid that evaporates when sprayed, with the intention of incapacitating a suspect when violent and fighting, or posing a risk to themselves or another.
DC –	Detective constable
DI –	Detective inspector
Door knocker –	Conmen who pray on the elderly or vulnerable, often hoping to take their antique/valuable items from them for a cheap price
DS –	Detective sergeant
DV –	Domestic violence

EDT –	Emergency duty team
Eyeball –	Got an eye on the target or suspect
Fatacc –	Fatal accident. It's not an acronym, it's Fat (for fatal) Acc for accident. Dogacc is an accident involving a vehicle and a dog. Polacc – an accident involving a police vehicle. Seracc – a serious accident involving more than two vehicles and where there may be serious injuries or damage.
FLO –	Force liaison officer, or family liaison officer
Gaoler –	The officer who assists the custody sergeant in the cells
Guv, boss, sir, ma'am –	Someone of the rank of inspector or higher
Handbagger, bagger –	Handbag thief
IC –	Codes to describe ethnicity of suspect
IC1 –	A white-skinned European
IC2 –	A dark-skinned European
IC3 –	Negroid types (light or dark skinned)
IC4 –	Indian or Pakistani types
IC5 –	Chinese, Japanese, inc others
IC6 –	Arabian, Egyptian types
Juvey –	A young person who came to the notice of the police
A job –	Something police respond to, could be 999 or crime report, or anything that you are dispatched to attend. Not to be confused with 'the job' – catch-all term for the Police Force, e.g. 'Is he in the job?' Or, 'Is she job?'
JPU –	Juvenile Protection Unit
Kwik-cuffs	
LIO, Collator –	Local intelligence office/officer
Misper –	Missing person
MOP –	Member of the public
Mounties –	Mounted branch
Obs –	Observations, watching and waiting and recording events, people, suspects
Old sweat –	Name for an officer with a fair bit of service, who knows the ropes, been there and done it fifty times

	over, seen many policy changes come and go and come back again, often PC or PS
OTS –	'Out taking statements', often said to wives or partners when they rang the station to speak to their other halves and they weren't there. Also known as 'over the side', especially in the CID office as some detectives would take a day off work to spend it with another person and not tell their partner. If someone wasn't in the office we never said someone was off duty; it always had to be 'out taking statements'. Could get quite tricky.
Paedophile, Paedo –	A person who commits sex offences on children including child porn
PC –	Police constable, the starting rank of all officers
Ped X –	Pedestrian crossing
Perve, Pervert etc –	Someone who comes to notice for sex offences, or lascivious behaviour
Pickpocket, dipper –	Someone who stole from pockets or bags
Plonk, Doris, Miss –	Old-fashioned terms for policewomen
PNC or CRO –	A check on the police national computer database to find out if someone has a criminal record. Better known by employers as CRB checks, which are carried out for certain jobs such as for those working with children or vulnerable people.
Polacc –	Police vehicle accident (vicinity only polacc – in the presence of a police vehicle but not involving the police vehicle)
Refs –	Refreshment break
Relief shift –	Officers working together as one team at the same time, under the same supervisory officers
Rent Boy –	A male, usually a juvenile, who loiters for the purposes of prostitution and who commits sex acts for payment
Shifts	
ET –	Early turn, 6 a.m.–2 p.m. or 7 a.m.–3 p.m.
LT –	Late turn, 2 p.m.–10 p.m. or 3 p.m.–11 p.m.

ND –	Night duty, 10 p.m.–6 a.m. or 11 p.m.–7 a.m.
SO –	Station officer
SOCO –	Scenes of Crime Officer. Usually civilian employees who are trained in forensics. They take photographs of injuries, accidents, bodies etc. They analyse a scene of crime for fingerprints, blood, DNA, and much more. As scientific advances become more complex their job is invaluable in the detection of crime.
SOS –	Street offences squad
SS –	Social services
Street person, tramp, vagrant, down and out –	Person living on the street
TDA or TWOC –	(Taking and Driving Away, or Taking Without Owner's Consent) Stealing a car, taking and driving away, taking without owner's consent
10/9 –	Urgent assistance
TI –	Trainee investigator
Tom, hooker, tommy tucker, tart, whore –	Female prostitute
Van-draggers –	People who steal from the back of delivery vans
VDRS –	Vehicle defect rectification scheme, a ticket to a driver/owner of a vehicle that gave them fourteen days to fix a problem with their car or they would be prosecuted. A very good way of dealing with minor vehicle defects and avoiding court.
VPU –	Vulnerable Persons Unit

Acknowledgments

The first person I would like to thank is Scott Pack because without him this book wouldn't be possible. If our paths hadn't crossed and he hadn't taken a chance on me, I would never have written *Undercover Cop*. I will forever be grateful to him for giving me this opportunity.

A huge thank you to the Friday Project team – Alice Tarbuck, who kept me on the right tracks, Katie for the illustration – wow! and copy-editor Nicola, for understanding what I was meaning to say when I wrote clumsy sentences, and for making them better.

I would like to give thanks and gratitude to my amazing group of friends, and writing and reading friends, who have all endured my angst, been mentors, read my work, helped with suggestions, and for being so supportive when I thought I was writing rubbish. Thank you for believing in me. As I can't publicly thank them without blowing my cover, I trust they know who they are – TH, SY, JD, AH, KE, CS, HH, NDG, SQ, JP, LS, SC, JM, VR, JS, JW, A(H)H, KS. And of course, all my social networking friends on Twitter and Facebook, even if they don't realise who the real me is.

To dear friends no longer with us. Two of the very best officers. I won't forget you. DS. ES.

Kenny and the kids – thank you for allowing me the time and space to write, not just this book but ever since I started writing all those years ago. Thanks for all the interruptions and demands that took me away from the computer, bringing me back into the family fold, because those moments helped me to sit back down again and write some more. Life's been tough at times but we've seen it through, all of us together. Thank you.

To everyone who's ever walked with me, on the beat or otherwise. Without you I wouldn't have any stories to tell. Thank you for being part of it.